AN IMPORTANT MESSAGE
FOR ALL ALLERGICS:
THIS BOOK WILL HELP YOU—

- Negotiate the modern-day allergy obstacle course
- Maintain a rich, well-balanced diet
- Identify the foods containing your particular allergen
- Recognize the most unexpected sources of allergens—like envelope or postage-stamp stickum, aspirin, liquor, vitamins or soap
- And much, much more.

WITH OVER 400 DELICIOUS RECIPES,
RECIPES FOR ALLERGICS
IS THE DEFINITIVE COOKBOOK
FOR PEOPLE WITH ALLERGIES.

RECIPES FOR ALLERGICS

Billie Little

BANTAM BOOKS
TORONTO · NEW YORK · LONDON · SYDNEY

RECIPES FOR ALLERGICS
A Bantam Book / January 1983

ISBN 0-553-22538-3

Published simultaneously in the United States and Canada

PRINTED IN THE UNITED STATES OF AMERICA

O 0 9 8 7 6 5 4 3 2 1

In memory of my Mother—
the dearest allergic in the world—
and to Bill, my loving husband.

B.L.

ACKNOWLEDGMENTS

I am deeply indebted to my Mother, Myra May Haas, for her recipes, which she at one time published and for which she has received international acclaim . . . and much is owned to those companies that have allowed me to include recipes of various substitutes: The Borden Company (MULL-SOY), Loma Linda Foods (SOYALAC), Mead Johnson (NUTRAMIGEN and SO-BEE), The Chicago Dietetic Supply House (CELLU), El Molino Mills (various flours and CAROB POWDER), The Ener-G Company (JOLLY JOAN), Worthington Foods (SOYAMEL) and Nu Vita Foods (SOYA CAROB).

I am very grateful to Doctor James W. Willougby of Kansas City., for himself and Doctor Herbert J. Rinkel (deceased), who has graciously granted me permission to use subject matter of their composition. Also their publisher, Charles Thomas, and, of course, to Velma Alcorn, Dietitian, for her assistance in checking for accuracy.

Then there is another list of those who contributed and to whom I own a debt of gratitude: **The Ladies Home Journal, McCall's Magazine, Good Housekeeping, Newark Evening** News, Los Angeles **Times** and others too numerous to list.

I cannot close this page without including a mention of the many, many hours and untiring efforts devoted by my collaborator, Dr. A. Chesmore Eastlake, who not only deserves my own enduring appreciation but that of all the allergics who will be helped by his abundant knowledge, which he has shared with us all.

The Author

CONTENTS

FOREWORD

In the days when the medical science of allergy was in its infancy, my mother suffered from hay fever, which was commonly thought at the time to be caused only by inhalation of something such as pollens or dust. While consulting a pioneer allergist she was found to be allergic to some foods as well and started to starve with an elimination diet much like diabetics had to do before insulin was discovered. Soon, however, Mother began to experiment with substitute foods, eventually compounding them into tantalizing recipes with all the food values of previously eaten foods, but without the poisonous effects.

Mother's recipes are included in this book, recipes that have truly stood the test of time! There are many other recipes also, some made with wonderful commercially prepared food substitutes not available in the "good old days."

If you are one of the 20,000,000 Americans suffering from a major allergy, suffering with unexplained tiredness, headaches, stomachaches, itches or loss of libido, you owe it to yourself to spend minutes a day trying these recipes section by section for a few weeks to see if you can find a cure for your miseries.

The Author

INTRODUCTION

This book is a combination of a primer on allergy for the layman, written by Doctor A. Chesmore Eastlake, and a simple compilation of tested recipes to be used by people who are allergic to certain foods. The vast majority of food-allergic people are allergic to corn, wheat, milk and eggs. The importance of these foods is related to the frequency of their use in pure form, not only daily but in almost every meal of every person, and also to the almost unbelievable extent that these foods are used in combination with other foods. When one is allergic to milk, the possibilities of contact with milk seem innumerable as compared to the few sources of contact with strawberries.

Many of the recipes found in one part of this book may be used in conjunction with those in another part, meaning that some of the recipes listed under "no egg" also contain "no corn" or "no milk," etc. To repeat all of the "no egg" recipes in other applicable parts of the book would make the book too large, so we have mentioned the recipe by section number when the recipe appears elsewhere. For example: In Part 4, NO CORN, NO WHEAT, the Apple Stuffing recipe appears in full and it is also referred to in Part 15 with just the name of the recipe and section in which it can be found. This also indicates that the recipe can be used as a NO CORN, NO WHEAT dish as well as a NO WHEAT dish.

In order to assist the allergic to avoid recipes containing the food or foods that give him trouble, the principal offenders, corn, eggs, milk and wheat, are capitalized throughout the book so one can more easily eliminate those recipes that one should not use.

A good deal of information about how to cook (such as how to buy and use which cut of meat) is omitted from this book, since the great majority of those persons interested in delving deeper into their health, or that of their loved ones, are already "good cooks."

A discussion of miscellaneous food allergies is included in the latter part of the book; and should be read first—before trying any of the recipes—because "miscellaneous foods" are used throughout the book and can be unsuspected sources of trouble.

A PRIMER FOR ALLERGICS

"We are what we eat" is as true today as it was 5,000 years ago when a Chinese sage said expectant mothers should not eat fish or chicken because these foods might cause skin ulceration. Three thousand years ago a Greek thought that people should choose food very carefully because a food customarily eaten once daily could cause serious problems if eaten twice in a day. Just before the birth of Christ another said: "One man's meat is another man's poison." So food allergies have been known for perhaps as long as man has existed.

There are many, many ways in which allergy may show itself in the body. Every cell, every tissue, every organ, every system—even the whole body, meaning life itself—can suffer from an allergy. Most allergies are easily recognized such as hay fever (better called allergic rhinitis), asthma, hives and eczema. Many other conditions are, or may be, of allergic origin. Some of these conditions include arthritis, urethritis, colic and headaches. A list of symptoms, disorders and diagnoses that may be of allergic origin in the broadest sense, follows:

acne
adrenalitis
alveolar proteinosis
anemia
angina pectoris
angio alveolitis
biliary colic
blepharitis
blood pressure, high or low
bronchitis
byssinosis
canker sores
angioedema
angioneurotic edema
aplastic anemia
arthritis
asthma
atopic dermatitis

bagassosis
bed wetting
berylliosis
dendritic ulcers
dental caries
dermatitis venenata
dermatomyositis
diarrhea
disseminated neurodermatitis
disseminated sclerosis
dizziness
eczema
edema
encephalitis
enuresis
eosinophilia
epilepsy
erythema
erythema nodosum
farmer's lung
fatigue
fever
cataracts
catarrh
chest and lung deformities
chilliness
collagen diseases
confusion
conjunctivitis
contact dermatitis
deafness
lichen urticarius
Loffler's syndrome
lupus erythematosus
lymph node swellings
maple bark disease
meibomitis
Ménière's disease
mental depression
migraine
multiple sclerosis
muscle aches
myasthenia gravis
nausea
nervousness
nettle rash
neurosis
night sweats
orchitis
otitis media
fibrillation of heart
fixed eruptions
flutter of heart
giant hives
Goodpasture's stain
granulocytopenia
hay fever
heart rhythm changes
hepatitis
hexamethonium fibrosis
histamine cephalagia
histiocytosis
hives
hydralazine syndrome
id
infertility
insomnia
keratoconus
sinus trouble
strophulus pruriginosa
sweating
tachycardia
thromboangitis obliterans
thyroiditis
tiredness
papular urticaria
periarteritis nodosa
photosensitivity
pleural effusion
premature contractions of heart
prostatic obstruction
pruritis ani
pulmonary arteritis
pulmonary hemosiderosis

purpura
rashes
regional ileitis
rheumatic fever
rheumatoid pneumoconiosis
salivary gland swelling
sarcoidosis
scleroderma
silicosis
ulcerative colitis
urinary burning
urticaria
uveitis
vomiting
warmth
Wegener's granulomatosis

Of course, most of the foregoing disorders have other causes than allergy including such diverse conditions as angina pectoris, cataracts and hepatitis, but all can be caused by an allergy. Probably any of the conditions may be caused by a food allergy specifically, although not all have been proved so to date. Some of the conditions listed, although acting like allergic disorders, and indeed the result of hypersensitivity or autoimmune reactions, cannot be helped by allergic means and some cannot be helped by any kind of treatment at the present time.

People may be allergic to any one of many of "100,000 things"—foods, pollens, house dust, fabrics, animals, bacteria, fungi, paint, perfume, drug chemicals, plastics, food additives, yeast in the morning toast—anything that one can think of—anything that one can touch, breathe, eat or have injected into him.

Contact allergens are the things that we touch, thousands of things such as poison ivy, wool, chemicals, cosmetics, pollens and dust.

Inhalant allergens include the things that we breathe into our bodies. These include dust and pollens again, animal danders, chemical fumes, feathers and fungi. These are also called airborne allergens.

Ingestant allergens are substances that enter our bodies through the mouth. Normally these are food and drugs; abnormally, especially in children and pregnant women, many other things may be listed as ingestants.

Injected antigens are drugs and vaccines. Insect stings might well be in this list also.

Some of the words related to allergy that one might hear, and want to know the meaning of, are defined here:

ALLERGY: An acquired ability to react to something in a way that a "normal" person would not react.

ANTIGEN: A substance which, when introduced to the body by any route whether by the skin, the mouth, the respiratory tract or by injections, will cause the formation of antibodies in susceptible (allergic) people. This is also called an allergen.

ANTIBODY: A substance produced in the body in response to the stimulation of an antigen.

SHOCK ORGAN: The tissue or organ involved in an allergic reaction.

HYPERSENSITIVITY: Or sensitivity, loosely used to mean the same thing as allergy—an increased ability beyond that of a "normal" person to react in an abnormal way.

HYPOSENSITIZATION: A process of reducing the severity of an allergy. This process is usually carried out by eating a very small amount of a food to which one is allergic and then gradually eating more and more of it at prescribed intervals until the body is used to it or by injecting increasing amounts of an antigen. Hyposensitization is sometimes wrongly called desensitization. Another word for hyposensitization is hypoimmunization.

The antigen-antibody reaction affects the shock organ(s) of an allergic person to produce his characteristic symptom(s) after a certain chain of events. First, one must come in contact with a substance that his body does not like. Against this foreign substance his body forms an antibody that becomes fixed to the shock organ. Then upon reexposure to the specific antigen, the specific antibody unites with the antigen. This causes a release of a chemical or chemicals that may be histamine or serotonin and these chemicals exert an effect on the shock organ to produce the allergic reation. If the shock organ is the lung, then asthma may result; if it is the nose, then allergic rhinitis (hay fever) may result.

Why this antigen-antibody reaction occurs, why it picks on certain people in a family, why it chooses a certain shock organ(s), why food will cause asthma in one person and eczema in another and both in a third is not known, but we are working on it all the time.

Allergic reactions to a food or other substance may be delayed or may make themselves known immediately. A typical type of immediate reaction is one wherein a person eats strawberries and develops hives in a few minutes. A delayed reaction may be observed by one who drinks milk and then has diarrhea several hours later or gas all the next day.

There are many predisposing factors that may be used to determine the chances of who may become allergic. The first and most important thing in guessing who will become allergic is the family history. Practically all people who have an allergy have an ancestor with allergy. Of course, this may be the mother or the father, but many times it is an uncle or a grandmother. Often a person will not know that his uncle had an allergy and may therefore deny the possibility of allergy in his family. This may happen because the uncle's allergy was so mild that it was not recognized as an allergy. Many times we hear that the uncle always had catarrh or "sinus" or that the grandmother suffered from bronchitis and shortness of breath all of her life although she never smoked. Now we believe that the uncle in question probably had a mild allergic rhinitis and that the grandmother had asthma. Asthma comes in various degrees, it does not always manifest itself so severely that the person spends all of his time sitting up in bed gasping for air. Asthma sometimes only shows itself as a little wheeze with violent exercise.

There is often a marked difference in children of allergic parents regarding the development of allergies. In a large family one child may have many food allergies early in life while another child may develop only a few food sensitivities when older. Some children of allergic parents may show positive skin tests to allergens without ever showing any signs of allergy outwardly. Various studies have shown that with one allergic parent about 35% of the children will be allergic and if both parents have a major allergy about 65% of the children will be allergic. Although a certain number of children of allergic parents have positive skin tests without showing signs of allergy at the present, a very large number of them will in the next ten years. Some people think it is a good thing to test all children of allergic parents to see which ones will react to various antigens and then watch these children more carefully when new foods are added to the diet.

The earlier in life that one develops food allergies the more severe they usually are. Therefore it is important to control allergies in children as they develop. As a food is added to the diet and evidence of even mild allergy occurs, the time to do something about it is right then.

There is probably no difference between boys and girls as to which in a family will develop which kind of allergy nor how severe it will be. Both sexes are equally liable.

There is probably no difference in climate either as to whether one will more likely have asthma or a cold weather allergy.

Some people will move to a desert climate from the seacoast and be better, others will find the dry air dries out their lungs and they will be worse. People sometimes think the Eastern cold makes their allergies worse so they move to Southern California, and as only previous Southern Californians know, they complain of the cold here, too, even though the temperature may be 30°F. higher in Southern California in the winter. Cold is a relative thing. Most of the difference is whether people are happy where they are and to what they are allergic. If they do not like the middle of a big city, the open country may make them feel much better. If they are allergic to grasses, the sagebrush country may make them feel better. If they are allergic to eggs or milk or wheat, the place they live makes much less difference.

Too much alcohol or tobacco is not good for anyone and the more especially if one is allergic to the components of either. Sometimes people think they become intoxicated more readily with 86-proof bourbon than with 86-proof Scotch. Occasionally a severe allergy to corn may be found to account for those who feel bourbon treats them badly.

There are many other factors that play a part in food allergy. Sometimes a person can eat a food that has been cooked that he cannot eat in its raw form. The reverse may be true also. Sometimes a person may be mildly allergic to many foods. If he eats one or two of these foods he may not have a reaction, but if he eats several in one meal his allergy may bother him. Some foods are known to hardly ever cause an allergic reaction while others cause allergy in a large number of people. The serious offenders are listed later.

There is no laboratory test of note to aid in the diagnosis of food allergy except for the determination of the presence of a certain type of white blood cell called an eosinophil in the course of a complete blood count (CBC). If the eosinophils make up between four and fifteen percent of the total number of white blood cells, an allergy may be reliably suspected.

Many millions of people are allergic to one or many foods. The more foods to which one is allergic, the more fun one can have trying different recipes to satisfy his appetite and leave him with a new sense of well-being.

Certainly it is true that older children and adults suffer from untreated allergies and these must be vigorously treated to make for a happier, healthier life. Regarding any illness, however, prevention is always easier and better than a cure or relief. With this in mind we should concern ourselves with people from the day of their birth. It is the responsibility of the mother, the pediatrician or the family doctor to attempt to ward off each allergic symptom in the infant as it appears from the first day of life until the individual is old enough to care for himself. Too many times we see a child of five, ten or fifteen years old who has had an allergy from birth or from age six months, starting perhaps as an eczema often dating from the introduction of cow's milk to the diet, which was never adequately treated. Now the child has polyps in his nose, hay fever, asthma and possibly even irreversible emphysema to ruin his whole life. The following notes are directed then, to the infant via his mother and doctor.

A recent survey has shown that nearly one out of every four children has a major allergy and that half of these had not been treated. Of the half who were treated, many received treatment directed at the symptoms, called nonspecific treatment, rather than treatment directed at the cause of the allergy.

Nonspecific treatment means relief of the symptoms of a disorder rather than curing or eliminating the cause of the disorder. Taking aspirin to relieve the pain of sinusitis is relieving a symptom, taking an antibiotic to kill the organisms causing the sinusitis, and therefore the pain, is specific therapy.

Nonspecific treatment of various allergic disorders includes younger relatives of the older cortisone to treat all of the allergy symptoms of the whole body at one time and antihistamines that are supposed to do the same thing. "Cortisone" is not good for a long-term cure—because it has bad side effects in too many people—and the antihistamines just do not do enough for enough people. For asthmatics there are bronchodilators to make the bronchial tubes larger. These may be given by mouth, by smoke, by nebulization with a small or large machine, by rectum and by injection either just under the skin, in the muscle or in the vein. There are drugs to dry the nose in hay fever, salves to relieve skin itch and expectorants to thin secretions in asthma—capsules, pills, sprays, liquids, ointments—even adjustments to the spine—hundreds and hundreds of combinations.

Allergy in children usually shows itself by skin disorders, particularly eczema or by gastrointestinal reactions such as colic, vomiting or diarrhea. Children may even start bronchial asthma early. Too often asthma is passed off as a cold with bronchitis even though it "wheezes." Most likely when the infant wheezes the handwriting-is-on-the-wall. More and more troubles are pending, so the time to act is now, not six months or six years from now. Often it is said the infant will "outgrow" his allergies . . . Often it is said of a six-year-old that he will outgrow his allergies (now he has had them five and one-half years). Often it is said the twelve-year-old will outgrow his allergies (and now he has had them eleven and one-half years). His asthmatic chest is protruding almost beyond his chin. Perhaps this child has been receiving some pills and drops, but has he had a good specific investigation? Ask the majority of adults, say forty years old, appearing for the first time for an allergy workup, when in their lives their allergy first started and they usually say "I have had it as long as I can remember." It is well known that hardly half of infants with untreated asthma will outgrow it. Many who do outgrow it, in some years, are left with some permanent, if slight, incapacity. Others may have "only a little asthma" left, but it is a shame to see fifteen-year-old boys in high school who have to take corrective physical education because their "only a little asthma" will not allow them to play only a little basketball. Any amount of asthma causes some damage to the lungs with each attack.

The more important symptoms of allergy through childhood are skin disorders including eczema and hives, colic, vomiting and diarrhea, asthma, hay fever, croup, conjunctivitis, nose bleeds, intermittent loss of hearing, tonsillectomy and adenoidectomy, especially if the tonsils and adenoids tend to recur and have to be removed again. It had been said that three-quarters of removed tonsils come from the relatively few markedly allergic children. The infant should be treated as soon as he shows the first sign of allergy.

The first place to look for an allergen in an infant is his food. Today he is now subjected to foods other than mother's milk much sooner in life than in past years. It is true that he may suffer from things that touch him—his clothes for the most part—but these are easily identifiable and seldom cause trouble early in life, especially if they are washed and rinsed well. Eventually the infant may become allergic to cats or dust, but the effect of these is usually not seen for some years.

If the infant is now showing allergy for the first time it will be easy for the mother to list everything new in the baby's life in the past few days. If the allergy is well established then the mother must work a little harder to recall when the eczema or colic or asthma first started, when it was worse and then correlate the dates of the beginnings and the worsenings with the addition of new foods to the diet.

Sometimes the allergy will become worse with increase in frequency of use of foods from occasional to daily. The food most recently added before the allergy became worse or started is the prime suspect. Any food may cause allergy, but some are more frequently the cause than others. Sometimes a child will "discover" his own allergies. If there is some food(s) that he will not eat, force him carefully, he may be allergic to it.

The mothers of children born to families with a history of allergy should keep a little diet diary for all the children. The suggestion could be passed on to mothers by the doctor who delivered the baby or who will take care of it. Make the diary simple, keep it in the kitchen, make a listing of all the ingredients of foods that the baby eats. Maybe at first, particularly, the day will only say, "beef, green beans, milk," When foods become more complex it is good to list the manufacturer's name, too, because there are different ingredients used by different companies. Then someday if an allergy develops, it will be so easy to check back to see what was new when the first red spot appeared. Another important thing about a food diary is to show relationship of foods. If a child shows allergy to one food, he is more likely to show an allergy to a relative of that food than to one of a different family of foods. If a child shows an allergy to a particular food, the other foods in the same family can be singled out in advance to be avoided until a much later time in life. Food families are funny. For instance the word "nut" is found in many different families of foods. The peanut is of the legume family related to peas, lima beans, lentils, kidney beans, carob, licorice and some gums! The almond nut is in the plum family related to plums and prunes, cherries, apricots, nectarines and peaches. One family of "real nuts" includes black and English walnuts, hickory nuts and pecans while another has hazelnuts and chestnuts. Who would think that buckwheat is not related to wheat at all but to rhubarb and sorrel? Fish such as tuna and perch are entirely different from crustaceans represented by the crab and shrimp and mollusks like the oyster and abalone. Melons such as cantaloupe and watermelon are in the gourd family with pumpkin and squash. Beet sugar is related to spinach, cane sugar to wheat. Fruit sugar (fructose) is derived from fruit; it looks and tastes like sugar (sucrose) but has almost twice the sweetening power. It can be used in certain foods, beverages and cereals to replace ordinary sugar. (***Note:*** It has been found that fructose on occasion may cause diarrhea.) The potato family includes potatoes (but not yam), tomatoes, eggplants, red and green peppers, chilies and tobacco!

When an allergy develops in an infant and removal of the last food from the diet seems to make little difference and nothing else seems to be causing his difficulty, skin tests may be needed. Infants can be skin tested by three methods—scratch, intradermal and passive transfer. Skin testing in infants is less reliable than in older children but should be used without hesitation. Good results have been obtained with babies only three months old. The allergy must be stopped as soon as possible. Scratch tests are done first because they are weaker and will find the more severe allergens. Intradermal tests are then done using the allergens to which the baby has not reacted. These tests are ten to a hundred times more powerful so are not used for the allergens to which the baby is highly sensitive for fear of causing a temporary increase in the baby's symptoms.

Scratch tests are easily made by scratching the skin just enough to break through the outer protective layer of the skin while not deep enough to draw blood. Then a little drop of antigen is rubbed into the scratch. If the test is positive, that is if the patient reacts to the antigen, a "mosquito bite" forms at the site of the positive antigen varying in size depending upon the degree of the reaction. Intradermal tests require a little more skill but are easily done by the experienced hand. With these tests a small amount of the antigen is injected into the layers of the skin with a tiny needle. Again a positive test is determined by the development of a mosquito bite at the site of injection.

When a food or several foods have been placed under suspicion, they are eliminated from the diet one at a time or all together. When a number and variety of foods are removed from the diet, one must be careful to substitute other foods to maintain proper balance of carbohydrates, fats, protein, minerals and vitamins. For instance, if cow's milk has to be removed from a small baby's diet, a meat-base milk or soybean or goat's milk will have to be substituted; or if wheat is removed, ricc or oats can be used. If the allergy clears in a few days or even sooner, then it is obvious that thc causative allergen is in the list of eliminated foods. These foods can be added back to the diet one at a time at 10-14 day intervals until one causes the allergy. When this one, or sometimes more than one, is found it or they are eliminated from the diet for years. For some mothers it might be less of a hardship to eliminate only one food at a time for about a week. If there is no bettering of the allergy, the presently eliminated food can be returned to the diet and another is then removed for another week's trial.

If the eliminated food is a common one such as corn, wheat, milk or eggs, which are found in an extensive variety of prepared foods, recipes to substitute for these foods will be required since the average mother is almost but not quite enough of a dietician. Whatever prepared foods or mixes or "store bought" foods are used, it will always be necessary to check labels of boxes to see for sure what the contents are. In the text of the book are lists showing the more common contacts with corn, wheat, milk and egg. Many of the foods and supplements containing corn, for instance, will amaze you.

Once a child is found allergic to foods, all new foods added to the diet must be watched with an "eagle-eye" for several days to be sure they do not cause a reaction, however minor. It is better to add only one new food at a time because if allergy occurs, the culprit is easily identified. Always remember if the new food is a complex one, a mixture of foods, to note all of the ingredients—even some candy bars have many components.

There is a group of foods that is the most likely to cause allergies, meaning that more people react to these and the reactions are more likely to be severe. Some people are surprised to see beef in the list, but it is so commonly used as a meat food that it has to be included. The more dangerous foods are:

beef	fish	peas
cabbage	lettuce	pork
chocolate	milk	potato
coffee	nuts	string beans
corn	onion	tomato
eggs	peanuts	wheat

For a child who has already proved to be allergic, these foods should be added later in life than for a child who has demonstrated no allergies. For instance, a child with an allergic skin disorder who is fed cow's milk has a much greater chance of developing asthma than one who is breast-fed. Therefore, if the mother's milk is inadequate and the child is already developing signs of eczema, a meat base or soybean base milk may well be used for the formula rather than cow's milk.

A word regarding children from the first day of their lives—the development of a normal range emotional pattern must be fostered with great care in a child ill with any disorder, but particularly in a chronic disorder. Regardless of the method used to detect a food allergy, the child must be treated as much as possible as if he were normal in every respect. Emotional wrecks are easily created by mishandling the child, if he is treated as a "sickly one," pitied, carried, overly protected, isolated, made to wear more clothes or different clothes than called for or singled out for special favors. If it had to be one or the other, it might be better for a child to be somewhat short of breath from asthma at age twenty rather than to be a confirmed "spoiled brat."

There is absolutely no doubt that food allergy occurs in millions of older children and adults. The numbers of these people affected is constantly disputed because their diets are now so complex that they may eat scores of separate food entities in a single week and because skin tests for foods are somewhat unreliable, at least compared to the skin tests for ragweed hay fever. Many times positive tests are found to foods that the particular person being tested rarely or never eats. Conversely, in the same person a negative test to milk may be obtained and yet he knows he had been allergic to milk for years because his nose starts to run within an hour after drinking a glass of milk or he may get severe stomach cramps in the same length of time.

There are many factors affecting the diagnosis of food allergy after the first years of life. Some of these are discussed here. There are different methods of extracting food antigens to make the material placed in the scratch or injected into the skin. Most foods are very complex chemicals. In the digestive tract foods are broken down into more simple chemicals for absorption into the body. Some people seem to make different combinations of these simpler chemicals for absorption than other people, and it is these particular combinations that cause allergy in the person in question. When the whole food is extracted to make the antigen, this person's particular chemical combination is not included and therefore he can have a negative skin test to a food to which he is allergic after his body has changed it.

People are different in other ways. Some react in a constant or fixed fashion to a food that reacts in them. This means that no matter when they eat the food or how much or even if they have not eaten the food for years, they will always react to it in their usual way. If this kind of person eats something to which he is highly allergic, such as shrimp, and even if a small amount is camouflaged in an onion dip he will feel his "throat being shut off."

Then there are other people who are allergic to a food in a cyclic or intermittent fashion that works in different ways. If a person of this nature eats a lot of his allergenic food for some days, as one would more likely do with milk than with papaya, he will begin to react to it. Then if he does not eat the food for a while his allergy tends to lessen and he can eat it again, if he is careful not to eat too much at one time.

Sometimes a person can eat a food in the wintertime and then in the summer he will react to it. This may suggest that he is allergic to something else, perhaps grass and/or weed pollen, and that it takes the combination of the two to produce an allergic reaction. Other things may influence food allergy such as cold or heat or drafts or even taking a bath that is just not the right temperature. (There are probably purely physical allergies, too, as witness the person who steps out into the bright sunlight and sneezes.)

Infections and emotions play a part also. Many times people think emotions cause allergic reactions. It is more likely that emotions trigger the gun loaded for allergy. If one removes the offending bullet (food) from the gun (the diet), then the emotional trigger will only click faintly in an empty chamber rather than setting off an explosion. If emotions caused allergy, then nearly everyone would have allergy.

Even more difficult to diagnose is the person who can tolerate very small amounts of a food every day of his life—such as the small amount of egg in the cookie he eats for an afternoon snack. But then one day he celebrates Sunday morning breakfast with a big omelet and his allergy celebrates. He may feel he is not allergic to egg because he has the false notion that if people are allergic to something, they are allergic to any amount of it. Pollen hay fever can work the same way; it may suddenly get bad enough to do something about in a summer following an unusually heavy spring rainfall that causes the grasses and weeds to shed more than the usual amount of pollen because of better growth.

Some other people seem to accumulate food in their bodies and finally react one day even without eating an abnormal amount that day. A baker may inhale flour for years and then begin to react to it.

When a person is allergic to more than one food his problem is more difficult but should never be thought of as insurmountable. To overcome the more complex allergy that many older children and adults have involves skin testing and a choice of dietary methods. A whole series of skin tests should be done to help rule in or out other allergies in addition to food allergies. Many of the antigens to which the patient reacts, or is suspected of being allergic to by history, are placed into a vaccine for hyposensitization and the series of injections is started. Most antigens put into a vaccine are those that cannot be seen and cannot be avoided because they are everywhere in the air such as pollens of trees, grasses and weeds and dust and molds that blow around easily. Allergens from many other things such as feathers in a pillow, horsehair in furniture, tobacco or a dog or cat are best avoided rather than placed in a vaccine for hyposensitization. Sometimes the pet of the eight-year-old has to be given a new life on the farm—someone else's farm—to save the life of the four-year-old.

All of the foods that are suspected of causing the person's allergy, again either by test or history, are eliminated to be reintroduced to the diet later perhaps. Hyposensitization injections for foods are much less reliable and even somewhat more dangerous than the injections against pollens and dust so that they are rarely given. Instead diet methods are used to determine which foods can be eaten with both gusto and good health.

Some doctors feel it is wise to complete as nearly as possible hyposensitization by all of the allergens that can be safely injected into a patient to get him as well as possible, if not actually totally relieved of his symptoms, before starting on what seems to be the more difficult treatment by diet. Of course, during this time bad foods are avoided and feathers and cats are removed from the environment.

Hyposensitization (or hypoimmunization) consists of a series of injections of a vaccine given subcutaneously (just under the skin) two or three times a week until the patient is well or as nearly well as possible. Some people need only six injections (shots) to be well, others may need a hundred. The average person needs about twenty-five.

Routinely, each succeeding injection consists of more of the active ingredients of the vaccine than in previous injections until the particular person's maintenance dose is reached. This maintenance dose is then given as often as necessary to keep the person as free of his symptoms as possible. The period between injections varies in different people—all the way from one injection every five days or so to one every month. One should probably never go beyond a month between injections.

The development of immunity to some diseases, such as smallpox, by injection is called an "active immunity" because something alive is injected. One shot of smallpox will last for many years. Injection of other substances that are not alive is called "passive immunity." Passive immunity lasts only a few weeks. An example of this is the use of gamma globulin against, say, hepatitis. A large, single injection of gamma globulin can be used because it is not a "foreign" substance to the body. Injections against an allergy are passive and since we do not want them to wear off in a few weeks, and they are foreign to the body, the body will become accustomed to them. Usually we start with something like one unit for the first dose, two units for the second, four for the third and so on until the maintenance dose may be as high as 5000 units and sometimes very much more. Five thousand units in the first dose would be very dangerous for the well-being of the highly allergic person.

Developing immunity to allergy by gradually increasing the dose "calluses" the body against the antigens much like developing calluses on your hands. If you take too large a dose of a shovel handle (the "allergen") at first, you will develop blisters, but if you use the shovel just a little more each time, three times a week, you will develop beautiful calluses (protection or immunity against the shovel handle).

There is "one shot per year" hyposensitization for allergy, but this has been used more for research than for general practice in the twenty-some-odd years of its existence, and it is not licensed for commercial manufacture by our government yet.

There are three more commonly used methods to test for food allergy besides the use of skin tests. These will be discussed in some detail to aid you in deciding how you want to go about ridding yourself of the tiredness, the headaches, the stomach aches, the itches or whatever else bothers you. All three methods require the use of a food diary to list the foods being eaten and to note reactions and when they occur.

The first method is very simple, but not too acceptable for most people, and it is little used although effective. The person eats nothing but meat, one kind of meat until his symptoms are relieved or becoming better at least. Some will try beef in different ways, some will use another meat. No spices, no gravies, no flavorings, just the meat. Two days will sometimes show a result, although hardly a complete cure so rapidly. We can live on meat alone for a long time because we are more carnivorous than herbivorous, and we are not going to run out of vitamin C and develop scurvy for a long, long time. Very soon add a carbohydrate, perhaps a potato or rye bread made without wheat, then a vegetable, then a fruit. If at any time a worsening of the allergy occurs the last food added should be dropped, maybe forever, and something else substituted for it. In time a good variety of foods can be eaten with very little hardship.

In a variation of this diet one eats nothing at all for two days much as some people do when starting a reducing diet. This clears the system in the majority of instances and then foods can be added, one at a time, with a few days interval between additions until bad foods are found and a good diet is established. If during the fasting period of two days the symptoms are not much relieved, one can suspect he might not have a food allergy after all.

The second method has been used for thousands of years although not in a scientific fashion until this century. The idea behind this method is to choose a well-rounded diet from foods other than those known to cause the most allergy in the most people. The more dangerous foods listed previously includes foods that should not be used. A list of foods that might be used for a good, well-rounded starting diet includes lamb, rice, sugar, canned pears and oatmeal. This diet is used exclusively for a period of time, usually about 10 days. If the allergy becomes better, then other foods, particularly the suspected ones, are added one at a time to the relatively few being eaten until a reaction does occur. If one is not better on the diet as originally started, then changes will have to be made in it before something else can be added.

It does take a long time to determine allergy to foods by this method unless one is very lucky to hit on the right things early in the series of tests. It is also rather difficult when eating out to always be sure of obtaining the particular food on your diet list, if it is different from the list above. Many times the diets seem rather monotonous and unsatisfying.

The third method requires the person to list all the foods he rarely eats or better has not eaten in the previous two months. Sit down for a few minutes, or walk through a market with pencil and paper looking at all of the fruits and vegetables, all of the canned goods, all of the various kinds of meat, and list those which have not been in the menu for a while. Some people eat only beef, that there is lamb and mutton, pork, rabbit and various fishes in the meat section sometimes surprises them. From this list of rarely eaten foods a great variety of foods can be chosen to make nourishing meals. Perhaps this method allows more leeway in selection when eating out, since one is not tied down to one or two meats, perhaps, but several. It is really best, however, to limit oneself to two of everything for a short while to make it easier to identify an unsuspected allergen. If one selects this method and makes his list of rarely eaten foods, it will still be good to use foods not included in the "bad list."

One thing that strikes you about this method is that if one is allergic to foods, it has to be to a food that he is eating much of the time, thus when the foods he eats are eliminated the allergy should go with them.

Regardless of the method chosen, one must prepare foods much as if one had "ulcers" to avoid allergens that may be hiding in something like sauces. (It could well be that if all of us "ate to live" rather than "lived to eat," that is if we ate less and more plainly, that we would have less gas and less fat on our bodies, both of which are only good for buoyancy in swimming.) The average person living to seventy years spends five years of his life just eating.

When one on a restricted diet eats at home he may make a gravy out of the meat juices and vegetable juices on his diet list, but when he eats out he should ask that the chef prepare his foods with nothing added. If one is on a wheat-free diet, he surely must not have some wheat flour added to his gravy, nor should he have his veal chop dipped in cracker crumbs, which usually contain wheat. Order à-la-carte. You can find restaurants that will alter their cooking slightly for you.

There may, however, be a few people so allergic to foods that they should train themselves for employment that will not require extensive traveling, employment that will allow them to eat mostly at home or to "brown sack" their lunch to work. If you have to go to a hospital the dietician can and will, in most instances, prepare foods within your diet limits.

Remember no one food is indispensable, perhaps no group of

foods. For instance some people eat no meat at all and seem to thrive.

When one person in the family is on a restricted diet, limited to perhaps two meats, two fruits, two vegetables, it is easy for the other members of the family to follow the same diet to make the cooking problems less for mother. Some things can be added for the other members of the family rather easily, if necessary, but basically all can eat the same foods.

People who are allergic to foods will often have to eat at home before going to a party because often "party foods" are not on their lists. There is no reason to be embarrassed about this in this enlightened age. Quite often if one takes the initiative one will find there are others who will have to do the same thing because of their own disorders. One cannot eat things too salty because of heart trouble, the second cannot eat peppery things because of his ulcers, a third will hardly eat a thing because she is trying to lose weight. At a small party with old friends this is less of a problem because the hostess knows the restrictions of all of her guests. On a camping trip or picnic you can always take your own foods.

Finding the foods to which you are allergic may take a lot of time, maybe even a whole year. A little reflection, however, will allow you to decide that after suffering for, say, thirty years now with various unhappinesses of food allergy and facing another fifty years of the same thing, the year or so to discover the cause of this distress will eventually seem to be a very short while—a fifty-year, paid-up health insurance policy in one year. If one has to eliminate a few tasty morsels forever, improved health will more than make up for them. Besides one will find these recipes so tasty that he will never miss the foods that bothered him.

Diabetics can live without pie and candy, you can live without wheat and fish—and you will not need a daily injection either.

A. Chesmore Eastlake, M.D.
Torrance, California

One-time Assistant Professor of Medicine, University of Oregon Medical Center, Portland Oregon, and
Faculties of:
Columbia-Presbyterian Medical Center, New York, N.Y.

University of California Medical Center, San Francisco, California
University of Colorado Medical Center, Denver, Colorado
Consultant United States Public Health Service Immigration Program

SECTION I

CORN ALLERGY

INTRODUCTION

A great number of allergists believe that corn is now the cause of more food allergy problems than any other item in the diet. In the last three decades corn has been used increasingly in a wide variety of foods and other products, so that now it is very difficult to avoid contact with corn in one form or another. We always say "read the label," but there are no laws to force a statement of the source of all food derivatives.

Sugar from corn may cause trouble for some people, whereas sugar from cane, beet or fruit may not. A cooking fat may state on the label that it is of vegetable composition only, with no animal fat included, but the source of fat, or oil, may be corn, olive, avocado, peanut, soy or cottonseed, making elimination of a specific food difficult.

Corn may bother people by inhalation of fumes such as popcorn, by contact with a corn-containing substance like talcum powder, and most commonly by simply eating corn. Sometimes one can tolerate corn in one form but not another. However, if one is allergic to corn in any form he must be careful with other contacts, because he will likely become allergic to all forms.

It is sad, but too often true, that when one is allergic to any of the cereal grains—corn, wheat, rye, oats, rice or barley—he may eventually become allergic to the other cereal grains one by one. Sometimes the onset of a reaction may be delayed for a long time by using smaller amounts of a grain than one would normally, and switching from one grain to another. If all cereal grains seem to cause trouble, then the carbohydrate in the diet will have to come from other sources, such as potato or fruit, and cooking oils or fats may have to be of animal origin such as rendered beef suet.

When one knows he is cereal-grain sensitive, he would best be careful about certain less obvious things than a piece of bread. He must be careful about flouring and breading of meats, and of sauces and gravies that are thick. Corn sugar is in "everything"—candy bars, canned fruits, etc., and may be in anything marked glucose or dextrose, sugars usually known for their "quick energy."

Throughout the parts devoted to corn the book emphasizes use of corn-free oil and corn-free sugar, that is, use oils and sugars made from other plants. Actually in both oil and sugar there is very little of the corn antigen remaining, so little that it would affect only the few very highly corn-allergic people. Cornstarch on the other hand is not nearly so pure. We have all seen people really allergic to beer and other alcoholic beverages! Finally, one must remember that "pure grain flours" are often contaminated with other grains. Check and be sure! A comprehensive list of corn contact follows. This list should be learned by corn-sensitive people.

Corn is found in the following:

- Adhesives
  - Envelopes
  - Stamps
  - Stickers
  - Tapes
- Ale
- Aspirin and other tablets
- Bacon
- Baking mixes:
  - Biscuits
  - Doughnuts
  - Pancake mixes
  - Pie crusts
- Baking powder*
- Batters for frying:
  - fish, fowl, meat
- Beers
- Beets, Harvard
- Beverages, carbonated
- Bleached wheat flours**
- Bourbon and other whiskeys
- Breads and pastries
- Cakes
- Candy
  - Box candies, all grades
  - Candy bars
  - Commercial candies
- Carbonated beverages
- Catsups
- Cereals
- Cheeses
- Chop suey
- Coffee, instant
- Confectioners' sugar
- Cookies
- Cough syrups
- Cream pies
- Cream puffs
- Cups, paper
- Custards

Dates, confection
Deep-fat frying mixtures
Dentifrices
Envelopes, gum on
Excipients or diluents in
- Capsules
- Lozenges
- Ointments
- Suppositories
- Tablets
- Vitamins

Flour, bleached**
Foods, fried
French dressing
Frostings
Fruits
- Canned
- Frozen

Fruit juices
Frying fats
Gelatin capsules
Gelatin desserts
Glucose products
Graham crackers
Grape juice
Gravies
Grits
Gums, chewing
Gummed papers:
- Envelopes
- Labels
- Stamps
- Stickers
- Tapes

Gin
Hams
- Cured
- Tenderized

Harvard beets
Holiday type stickers
Ices
Ice Creams
Inhalants
- Bath powders
- Body powders
- Cooking fumes—fresh corn
- Popcorn
- Starch
- Starch while ironing
  - Starched clothes
  - Talcums

Jams
Jellies
Leavening agents
- Baking powders
- Yeasts

Liquors
- Ale
- Beer
- Gin
- Whiskey

Meats
- Bacon
- Bologna
- Cooked, with gravies
- Ham, cured or tenderized
- Lunch ham
- Sausages, cooked
- Wieners (frankfurters)

Milk, in paper cartons
Monosodium glutamate
Oleomargarine
Paper containers:
- Boxes
- Cups
- Plates
- (these three only when foods have a moist phase in contact with these cartons)

Pastries
- Cakes
- Cupcakes

Peanut butters
Peas, canned

Pies, creamed
Plastic food wrappers (the inner surfaces may be coated with cornstarch)
Powdered sugar
Preserves
Puddings
Rice
  Coated
Salt
  Salt cellars in restaurants
  Salt seasoning
Salad dressing
Sandwich spreads
Sauces for:
  Meats
  Fish
  Sundaes
  Vegetables
Sausages, cooked or table-ready
Sherbets
String beans
  Canned
  Frozen
Soups
  Creamed
  Thickened vegetable
Soybean milks
Sugar, powdered
Syrups, commercially prepared
Talcums
Teas, instant
Toothpaste
Tortillas
Vanillin
Vegetables
  Canned
  Creamed
Vegetables, frozen*
  Peas
  String beans
Vinegar, distilled
Vitamins
Whiskeys
  American brandies, both apple and grape, bourbon and "scotch"
Wines, American
  Dessert
  Fortified
  Sparkling
Zest

*Read labels—if in doubt, write the manufacturer.
**Most all flour is pure bleached wheat flour, but check the label!

PART 1

No Corn

(NOTE: Be sure to use soy margarine in all corn milk recipes where margarine is called for. Baking powders and sugars should all be corn-free brands.)

APPETIZERS

ANCHOVY PASTE ON POTATO CHIPS

Thin potato chips
Corn-free margarine
1 (2-ounce) can anchovies
2 tablespoons chicken fat or olive oil

Lightly brown potato chips in margarine. Mash anchovies with fork. Mix thoroughly with chicken fat or olive oil. Spread lightly on potato chips.
Makes approximately ¼ cup.

BREADS

(*NOTE: All flours, baking powders, and oils should be corn-free.*)

GRAPENUT BREAD

1 cup Grapenuts
2 cups sour MILK
4 cups FLOUR
¾ cup cane, beet or fruit sugar
1 teaspoon baking soda
1 tablespoon baking powder
½ teaspoon salt
2 EGGS

Let the grapenuts stand in the milk while you get the other ingredients ready. Grease 2 5x9x3¼-inch loaf pans with corn-free fat. Sift flour, sugar, soda, baking powder and salt. Add one egg to half the flour mixture, and beat until smooth; beat in remaining egg and grapenut-milk mixture, then rest of flour mix. Bake at 350°F. for 35 minutes. Makes 2 loaves.

NUT BREAD

2 EGGS
1½ cups MILK
1 teaspoon salt
4 teaspoons corn-free baking powder
2 cups FLOUR
2 cups graham FLOUR
1 cup cane, beet or fruit sugar
1 cup nuts finely chopped*

Grease 2 loaf pans with corn-free fat. Beat eggs and add to milk. Mix all the dry ingredients and combine well with the liquid. Pour into the loaf pans and let rise for 20 minutes in a warm place, then bake for 1 hour in a 300°F. oven. Remove from pans and butter crust with corn-free spread. Makes 2 loaves.

*In all recipes use only nuts you are not allergic to.

RICE MUFFINS

4 cups rice FLOUR
4 teaspoons corn-free baking powder
2 teaspoons salt
1 cup cane, beet or fruit sugar
2 EGGS
1½ cups water and 1½ cups Soyalac liquid, combined
2 tablespoons corn-free margarine, melted

Sift dry ingredients. Combine eggs, water-Soyalac mixture and shortening. Add to dry ingredients and stir just enough to combine. Fill greased muffin pans about ½ full. Bake at 400°F. for about 25 minutes. Makes 2 dozen.

BANANA BREAD

1 cup cane, beet or fruit sugar
½ cup BUTTER
2 EGGS
2 bananas, crushed
3 tablespoons SOUR CREAM
1 teaspoon baking soda dissolved in a little milk
2 cups FLOUR
1 cup nuts
½ teaspoon vanilla

Cream sugar and butter. Add the unbeaten eggs. Then beat in bananas, sour cream, baking soda, flour, coarsely chopped nuts and vanilla. Pour into greased pans. Bake at 350°F. for about 1 hour. Makes 1 large or 2 small loaves.

DATE-NUT BREAD

1 cup chopped dates
½ cup chopped nuts
1 cup hot water
¼ cup BUTTER
¾ cup brown sugar or beet sugar
1 EGG
½ teaspoon salt
1½ cups potato flour
½ cup graham FLOUR
1 teaspoon baking soda

Soak dates and nuts in the hot water and let stand while preparing butter mixture. Cream butter with sugar. Add the egg and beat well. Sift dry ingredients except for soda. Add soda to the date mixture, then combine with sifted mixture. Pour into a loaf pan that has been greased and floured with corn-free fat and flour. Bake at 350°F. for 45 minutes. Makes 1 large loaf or 2 small loaves.

*ROLLS

- **1 cup MILK**
- **1 cake compressed corn-free yeast**
- **¼ cup cane, beet or fruit sugar**
- **¼ cup BUTTER**
- **1 cup warm mashed potatoes**
- **2 EGGS, beaten**
- **Corn-free flour**
- **Salt**

Scald the milk and soak yeast. Add sugar, butter, potatoes and then the eggs to the scalded milk. Stir in sufficient flour (up to 1 cup) to make a sponge and let rise until light. Add salt and enough flour to make a firm dough. Let rise until doubled in bulk. Shape into rolls and let rise. Bake at 450°F. for about 10 to 12 minutes. Makes 2 dozen small rolls.

CARAMEL ROLLS

- ***Rolls (recipe above)**
- **2 cups confectioners' cane, beet or fruit sugar**
- **1 tablespoon BUTTER, melted**
- **½ teaspoon mapleline (similar to maple extract)**

Use above recipe and refrigerate. Roll dough into a 6x12-inch rectangle, ½ inch thick. Cut into 1-inch slices and arrange in a buttered pan. Let rise until doubled in bulk. Bake 15 to 20 minutes at 450°F. Combine sugar, butter and mapleline with enough water to make it spreadable. Top rolls with icing while warm. Makes 2 dozen small caramel rolls.

QUICK COFFEE CAKE

- **½ cup cane, beet or fruit sugar**
- **1 generous tablespoon BUTTER**
- **1 EGG**
- **½ teaspoon cinnamon**
- **¾ cup MILK**
- **2½ cups corn-free flour**
- **2 teaspoons corn-free baking powder**
- **Pinch of salt**

Combine all the ingredients and pour into 8x8x2-inch pans that have been greased with corn-free oil. Put a mixture of butter, sugar and cinnamon on top. Bake at 350°F. for about 20 minutes. Serves 6 to 8.

BISCUITS, APPLE STYLE

- **4 tablespoons BUTTER**
- **1 EGG, beaten**
- **1 cup MILK**
- **2½ cups sifted potato flour**
- **3½ teaspoons corn-free baking powder**
- **½ teaspoon cinnamon**
- **1 cup plus 2 tablespoons beet, cane or fruit sugar**
- **½ teaspoon nutmeg**
- **1 cup chopped apples**

Mix butter, egg, milk and dry ingredients (except for 2 tablespoons sugar and the spices) together. Pour apples over all. Form into small biscuits and place on cookie sheets. Combine the remaining sugar and spices and sprinkle over biscuits. Bake at 350°F. for 20 minutes. Makes 5 dozen small biscuits.

BUTTERMILK SCONES

- **2 cups potato flour**
- **1½ teaspoons beet, cane or fruit sugar**
- **1 level tablespoon corn-free baking powder**
- **½ teaspoon baking soda**
- **¼ teaspoon salt**
- **4 rounded tablespoons BUTTER**
- **1 EGG, beaten**
- **1 cup BUTTERMILK**

Combine dry ingredients and work in butter. Add egg to buttermilk and pour into dry ingredients. Roll to a ⅛-inch thickness and brush with melted butter. Cut into squares and fold over into triangles. Place in a dish that has been greased with corn-free fat. Bake at 450°F. for about 15 minutes. Makes about 3 dozen.

SOUP

MARROW BALLS FOR SOUP

1 cup matzo meal
½ teaspoon baking powder
1 tablespoon grated onion
1 EGG, well-beaten
3 tablespoons marrow or chicken fat, melted
4 to 6 tablespoons soup stock or water (enough to make a stiff paste)
2 tablespoons chopped parsley
Salt to taste
Few grains of black pepper

Mix matzo meal, baking powder and onion. Add egg and marrow or chicken fat. Add soup or water, gradually stirring all the while. (The mixture must be stiff enough to hold together.) Add parsley, salt and pepper. Roll into tiny balls, the size of a marble. Refrigerate until ready for use. Just before serving, add the balls to the boiling soup and cook for 10 to 20 minutes. Makes 2 dozen small balls.

SALAD

JELLIED PEAR SALAD*

1 (No. 2) can sliced pears
1 (3-ounce) package lemon Jell-O
½ to 1 cup water
lettuce

Drain pears. Take juice and add sufficient water to total 2 cups liquid. Heat 1 cup liquid, mix with gelatin. Add balance of liquid, pour into 4-cup mold. When Jell-O is cooled and is slightly thickened, add sliced pears, chill. Unmold on crisp lettuce. Serves 4.

*If you want to use French dressing with this salad, mix together:
2 tablespoons vinegar (lemon or grapefruit juice)
6 tablespoons salad oil
1 teaspoon salt
⅛ teaspoon pepper (optional)
1 tablespoon sugar

DESSERTS

Cakes

LARGE CAKE

1 (18.5-ounce) box lemon cake mix.**
1 lemon pie filling mix
4 EGGS
⅔ cup peanut or safflower oil
⅔ cup hot water
Shavings of lemon peel

Put all ingredients in the mixer for 5 or 6 minutes at low speed. Bake in a Bundt pan in 350°F. oven about 40 to 45 minutes, or until brown. Remove cake from oven and let stand for 10 to 12 minutes then invert on a bottle neck. When completely cool remove from pan. About 16 servings.

**Check label

Candies

PRALINES (recipe in Part 6)

CATHIE'S CANDY DATES

1 cup MILK
1 tablespoon BUTTER
2 cups cane, beet or fruit sugar
½ to ¾ cup finely chopped walnuts
½ pound fresh dates

Heat milk and add butter and sugar. Cook to soft ball stage. Add nuts and dates, remove from fire and beat until the dates are pulverized and the candy is stiff. Roll in a damp cloth to dry and then cut in slices. Makes about 1½ dozen.

GEMS OF THE EAST

2 envelopes unflavored gelatin
½ cup cold water
¾ cup boiling water
2 cups granulated cane, beet or fruit sugar
Salt
Vegetable coloring (corn free)
Vanilla or other flavoring
Confectioners' cane, beet or fruit sugar

Soften gelatin in cold water. Combine boiling water, granulated sugar and salt, stirring until the sugar is dissolved. Bring to a boil. Add gelatin, and stir until dissolved. Boil slowly for 15 minutes then remove from heat, tint and flavor as desired. Pour into an 8x8x2-inch pan that has been rinsed in cold water. Let stand for at least 12 hours, or until firm (do not refrigerate). Using a wet knife, loosen candy from edges of pan, invert onto a board that has been sprinkled with sifted powdered sugar, and tap lightly to remove easily from pan. Cut into shapes and roll in powdered sugar. Serves 4 to 6.

WALNUT CLUSTERS

4 ounces sweet cooking chocolate
¾ cup broken walnuts

Chop chocolate and melt over boiling water, stirring constantly. Stir in walnuts and drop by tablespoons onto waxed paper. Chill. Makes 8 to 10.

PAULINE'S BUTTERSCOTCH DELIGHTS

1 (12 ounce) package butterscotch morsels
1 cup chopped pecans
1 (3 ounce) can "Chinese Noodles"

Melt ingredients together in top of double boiler. Drop by tablespoons on waxed paper and refrigerate. Makes 1 to 1½ dozen.

Pie

LEMON CAKE PIE

2 EGGS, separated
1 tablespoon corn-free flour
1 cup sugar
1 cup hot MILK
1 tablespoon BUTTER, melted
Juice and grated rind of 1 lemon
1 baked (but not browned) pastry shell

Beat egg yolks and add flour slowly, then sugar. Beat until smooth. Gradually add milk, butter, lemon juice and rind. Beat egg whites until stiff and fold in. Pour into the pie shell. Bake in a 300°F. oven for about 25 minutes. When baked it will be puffy and resemble a sponge cake on top, a custard underneath. Serves 6.

Puddings

LEMON PUDDING

3 EGGS
1 cup cane, beet or fruit sugar
2 tablespoons corn-free flour
Pinch of salt
2 tablespoons BUTTER, melted
1 teaspoon vanilla
1 cup MILK
½ cup orange and lemon juice combined

Separate eggs and beat whites until stiff. Add sugar, flour and salt to yolks. Then add butter, vanilla, milk and juice. Fold in egg whites. Bake as custard in slow oven in a pan of water at 350°F. for about 1 hour. Serves 4 to 6.

APPLE CHARLOTTE

2 thick slices corn-free bread
½ teaspoon corn-free baking powder
1 teaspoon vanilla
¼ cup of nuts (pecans, or any that can be tolerated)
Handful of raisins
1 tablespoon BUTTER, melted
½ cup cane, beet or fruit sugar
6 apples
4 EGGS
Heavy CREAM (optional)

Squeeze bread slices (removal of crust optional) dry after soaking in water. Add baking powder, vanilla, nuts, raisins, butter, sugar, apples and 2 eggs. Separate remaining 2 eggs and add yolks. Bake in greased baking dish, at 350°F. for approximately 45 to 50 minutes, or until brown. Beat 2 whites stiff for a meringue (or add to the charlotte before baking and use whipped cream for a topping.)* Serves 4 or 5.

*Beat remaining whites very stiff, fold into charlotte mixture carefully. *(Note: If preferred, you may make a meringue with whites stiffly beaten, to which 3 tablespoons sugar have been added while beating.)*

CHOCOLATE BLANCMANGE

1½ cups MILK, scalded
4 tablespoons cane, beet or fruit sugar
1 ounce chocolate, melted
½ cup cold MILK
1 envelope gelatin
½ teaspoon vanilla
½ teaspoon salt

Mix scalded milk, sugar and melted chocolate. Pour cold milk in a bowl and sprinkle gelatin on top. Stir thoroughly. Add to hot mixture and stir until gelatin is dissolved. Cool slightly, then add vanilla and salt. Turn into 3 or 4-cup mold that has been rinsed with cold water and chill. When firm, unmold and serve with whipped cream. Serves 4 to 6.

PART 2

No Corn, No Egg

BREADS

YEAST BREAD

4 teaspoons sugar
1 cake yeast
1 scant cup tepid water
2 cups MILK, scalded
2 cups cold water
8 cups corn-free flour
2 teaspoons salt

Dissolve sugar and yeast in the tepid water, but do not let stand more than 10 minutes. Combine scalded milk and cold water and add to yeast mixture. Add half the flour, beat until smooth, then add the remaining flour and salt. Knead until smooth and elastic. Place in a greased bowl, cover and set aside in moderately warm place for about 2 hours. Mold into loaves. Place in well-greased bread pans (half full). Cover and let rise for one hour, or until doubled in bulk. Preheat oven to 400°F. then lower to 350°F. and bake for 40 to 50 minutes. Makes 3 loaves.

SWEET POTATO MUFFINS

1 cup mashed sweet potatoes
1 cup dry rolled oats and dry Soya meal combined
¾ cup hot water (poured over flours)
1 tablespoon baking powder
½ cup chopped nuts
1 teaspoon salt
3 tablespoons shortening, melted
2 tablespoons honey

Mix in order given. Place in well-greased muffin pans and bake for 20 minutes in a 400°F. oven. Makes 18.

ROLLED OATS BREAD

2 cups boiling water
1 cup rolled oats
½ cup molasses
2 teaspoons salt
1 tablespoon BUTTER, melted
1 cake yeast dissolved in ½ cup lukewarm water
Corn-free flour

Add boiling water to rolled oats and allow to stand for 1 hour. Add molasses, salt, butter and yeast. Add up to 1 cup flour slowly to make stiff dough. Knead well, then let rise. Knead again, very little. Divide into two bread pans and let rise again. Bake in a 350°F. oven for 40 minutes. Makes 2 loaves.

RYE ROLLS

1 cup potato flour
3 cups rye FLOUR
1 teaspoon salt
2 tablespoons baking powder
1 tablespoon shortening, melted
1½ cups MILK

Sift together dry ingredients. Add shortening and milk to make a soft dough. Knead on a floured board. Shape into rolls. Put into greased muffin pans and allow to stand in warm place for 20 minutes. Bake at 475°F. for 15 to 20 minutes. Makes 12.

BAKING POWDER BISCUITS

2 cups corn-free flour
4 teaspoons corn-free baking powder
1 teaspoon salt
2 tablespoons shortening
¾ to 1 cup MILK or water

Sift together dry ingredients. Rub in shortening with tips of fingers. Add milk, mix, using knife, until all is soft and easily worked, soft and light but not sticky. Turn out onto floured board. With floured hands, knead about 2 dozen strokes until smooth. Lightly roll to about ¾ ″ thickness. Shape with biscuit cutter. Put on ungreased cooking sheet (close together for softer biscuits, 1½″ apart for crustier ones.) Prick with knife tip, or fork. Bake at 450°F., 12 to 15 minutes. Makes 12 to 15.

DUMPLINGS

1 cup corn-free flour
½ teaspoon salt
3 teaspoons baking powder
6 tablespoons MILK

Sift together dry ingredients and add milk to make a soft dough. Drop by spoonfuls into hot stew and steam, covered, for 20 minutes. Makes 6.

SPAGHETTI

1 (12-ounce) box egg-free spaghetti
1 tablespoon salt
1 cup MILK
1 tablespoon BUTTER, melted
Croutons (use corn- and egg-free bread)

Cover spaghetti with boiling salted water and cook for about 9 minutes. Heat milk to boiling point, then add butter. Drain spaghetti. Pour hot milk over spaghetti. Meanwhile, have 2 slices of bread cut into ¾-inch squares. Brown in butter as croutons. Serve hot over spaghetti. Serves 8.

SPAGHETTI AND CHEESE

- **½ box egg-free spaghetti**
- **1 tablespoon salt**
- **1 cup hot MILK**
- **1 tablespoon BUTTER, melted**
- **2 ounces CHEESE**

Cover spaghetti with cold water and add salt. Cook from 9 to 15 minutes then drain. Combine milk and butter and pour over spaghetti. Cut cheese into bits and sprinkle on top. Brown under broiler. Serves 4.

PART 3

No Corn, No Milk

PUDDINGS

FROZEN STRAWBERRY PUDDING

1 quart strawberries
1 cup cane, beet or fruit sugar
½ pound macaroons
1 cup white wine
4 EGG yolks, beaten

Alternate sugared strawberries and macaroons in a pudding dish. Heat wine and pour gradually over yolks. When slightly cooled, pour over the berries and macaroons and mix. Freeze or fill an airtight mold and pack in ice and salt for 6 hours. Makes 1½ quarts.

BANANA FLUFF

1 cup boiling water
1 (3-ounce) package lemon gelatin (or 5½-ounce for double recipe)
3 or 4 ripe bananas

Add boiling water to lemon gelatin. Rub bananas through a sieve. Add to lemon gelatin and cool. When almost set, place bowl in pan of cracked ice or very cold water. Beat with eggbeater to a very stiff froth. Pile lightly into glasses. Serve at once, or chill until ready to serve. Serves 8.

TORTE

CRACKER TORTE

2 EGG yolks
1 cup cane, beet or fruit sugar
4 ounces bitter chocolate
1 teaspoon baking powder
8 soda crackers, crushed
1 teaspoon cloves, ground
1 (6-ounce) glass of whiskey
6 EGG whites, stiffly beaten
Lord Baltimore Frosting*

Cream the yolks and sugar. Melt chocolate over hot water, then add to egg mixture. Add baking powder, cracker meal, cloves and whiskey. Fold in egg whites. Pour into spring form pan greased with corn-free oil. Bake in a preheated 400°F. oven for 30 to 50 minutes. Ice with Lord Baltimore Frosting.

*Lord Baltimore Frosting, Part 13.

PART 4

No Corn, No Wheat

BREADS

RYE BREAD

- **1 cake yeast, crumbled**
- **¾ cup lukewarm water**
- **½ cup Sobee liquid**
- **2 tablespoons corn-free vegetable oil**
- **4 teaspoons cane, beet or fruit sugar**
- **1 teaspoon salt**
- **3 cups sifted rye FLOUR**

Dissolve the yeast in ¼ cup of the lukewarm water. Mix Sobee liquid to the remaining ½ cup lukewarm water with oil, sugar and salt. (All ingredients should be lukewarm.) Add the flour and beat until smooth. Turn out onto a floured board. Knead, adding flour as needed (up to ¼ cup) to keep dough from sticking. Knead until dough is smooth. Dough may be a little moist but should be workable, if handled lightly. Put into a bowl which has been greased with corn-free oil. Turn dough once to bring greased side up. Cover with a damp cloth and let stand in warm place (80°F. to 90°F.) until dough is doubled in bulk. To tell when dough has doubled, press deeply with fingers, then lift fingers. If holes do not close, it's ready to rework. Turn out on board and knead again for about 5 minutes. Shape dough into a smooth loaf. Place in a greased pan, grease top of loaf with soy butter or corn-free shortening, cover and let rise until doubled in bulk. Bake in a 375°F. oven for about 45 minutes, or until well browned. Makes 1 loaf.

ORANGE SOYBEAN BREAD

1 cup orange juice made from ⅓ cup juice plus finely chopped rind and pulp to total 1 cup
2 teaspoons liquid Cellu sweetening
3 tablespoons melted corn-free fat
3 EGGS, separated
½ cup Cellu soybean flour
1 cup Cellu washed rice bran
1 tablespoon Cellu baking powder
½ teaspoon salt

Combine orange juice and sweetening. Heat slowly in a small saucepan until fruit reaches the boiling point. Remove from heat and cool. To orange mixture add fat and beaten egg yolks. Combine thoroughly. Mix dry ingredients and combine with egg yolk and orange mixture. Stiffly beat egg whites and fold in. Pour into a loaf pan that has been lined with wax paper. Bake in a preheated 350°F. oven for 20 minutes. Then lower temperature to 325°F. and bake 15 or 20 minutes longer. Makes 1 loaf.

SWEET POTATO BREAD

2 cups sifted rice FLOUR
¾ cup corn-free sugar
1 tablespoon corn-free baking powder
1 teaspoon salt
¼ teaspoon mace
½ cup finely chopped pecans
2 EGGS, beaten well
1 cup mashed sweet potatoes
½ cup MILK
3 tablespoons BUTTER
6 or 8 pecan halves

Sift dry ingredients and stir in pecans. Blend together eggs, sweet potatoes, milk and butter. Add liquid to flour mixture and stir until blended. Turn into a greased 4x8-inch loaf pan and press pecan halves over top to form a design. Bake at 350°F. for about 1 hour and 10 minutes, or until straw inserted in center comes out clean. Cool about 10 minutes in pan before removing, then slice thinly. Makes 1 loaf.

RYE MUFFINS

- 1 cup rye FLOUR
- ¼ cup potato flour
- 1 level tablespoon corn-free baking powder
- ⅛ teaspoon salt
- 2 EGGS
- ¾ cup MILK
- 2 tablespoons BUTTER

Sift flours and baking powder. Add eggs, milk and butter. Mix well, then add to flour mixture. Preheat oven for 15 minutes. Bake in a 425°F. oven for 20 minutes. Makes 8 to 12 muffins.

SOYBEAN MUFFINS

- 1 EGG
- 1 level teaspoon salt
- 1 tablespoon BUTTER, melted
- 4 walnuts, broken in small pieces
- 1½ cups soybean FLOUR
- 2 level teaspoons corn-free baking powder
- ½ cup CREAM
- ½ cup water

Beat egg well. Add salt, butter and walnuts, stirring together. Combine flour and baking powder, then sift. Add alternately with egg mixture to cream and water. Pour into well-buttered, warm gem pans. Bake in a 450°F. oven for 15 to 18 or 15 to 20 minutes. Makes eight large or 12 to 14 small muffins.

SOYBEAN PANCAKES

- 3 EGGS
- ½ teaspoon salt
- ½ teaspoon baking powder
- ½ cup soybean FLOUR
- ½ cup MILK

Beat eggs well. Add salt. Combine baking powder and flour and add alternately with the milk to the eggs. Spread a spider* thickly with butter and keep in a cool place until needed. Bake 10 minutes in a 500°F. oven, then reduce heat to 350° and continue baking for another 5 minutes. Makes 8 to 10 pancakes.

*Ovenproof, cast-iron frying pan with short feet.

RICE WAFFLES

3½ cups rice FLOUR
2 tablespoons corn-free baking powder
2 teaspoons salt
3 cups MILK
4 EGG yolks, beaten
4 EGG whites, beaten
6 tablespoons BUTTER (or margarine), melted

Sift dry ingredients together, then add milk, beaten yolks and fat. Fold in stiffly beaten egg whites. Bake in hot waffle iron. Serve hot with butter and syrup. Makes 1 dozen small waffles.

WAFFLES

1½ cups rice FLOUR
2 cups potato starch
2 teaspoons salt
6 teaspoons baking powder
2½ cups MILK
4 EGG yolks, beaten
4 EGG whites, beaten
6 tablespoons BUTTER, melted

Sift dry ingredients, then add milk and beaten yolks and fat. Fold in stiffly beaten egg whites and bake in hot waffle iron. Makes 1 dozen waffles.

POULTRY STUFFING

APPLE STUFFING

1 teaspoon paprika
¼ teaspoon pepper
¼ teaspoon cinnamon
⅛ teaspoon cloves
1½ teaspoons salt
½ teaspoon celery salt
4 cups Swedish rye crumbs
½ cup BUTTER
1 cup boiling water
4 cups chopped apples
1 cup chopped celery
1 medium-sized onion, chopped

Mix seasonings and crumbs. Add butter to water with remaining ingredients. Mix all together. *Note:* Any or all spices may be omitted. Makes 11 cups stuffing.

VEGETABLES

EGGPLANT

1 eggplant
Rice or potato FLOUR
Soy butter or safflower margarine
1 onion, sliced thin
Pepper and salt to taste
Pinch of marjoram

Cut eggplant into thin slices. Soak in salted water to cover, weighted down with plate (eggplant will rise to surface if not weighted). Remove, wash and dry slices. Dredge in mixture of flour and salt. Melt soy butter or margarine and dip eggplant in shortening, turning to coat both sides. Then add the onion and seasonings. Place in baking pan and bake in a 400°F. for 15 minutes or until tender. Turn once when bottom is brown. Serve very hot. Serves 4.

COOKIES

CHOCOLATE MACAROONS

1 pound almonds
2 ounces Baker's chocolate
1 pound confectioners' sugar (cane, beet or fruit)
2 level teaspoons arrowroot
8 EGG whites, beaten

Mince almonds very fine. Grate chocolate. Add sifted sugar, arrowroot and egg whites. Drop batter by teaspoon into a damp hand. Roll. Drop on buttered cookie sheet. Bake in a preheated 425°F. oven for 15 to 20 minutes, or until slight crust forms. Allow to get cold before removing from cookie sheet. Makes about 3 dozen.

MACAROONS

1 EGG
½ cup cane, beet or fruit sugar
¼ teaspoon vanilla
⅔ cup rolled oats
Pinch of salt
⅓ cup chopped walnuts
2 teaspoons BUTTER, melted

Beat egg until very light. Add sugar slowly, beating constantly. Add vanilla, oats, salt, nuts and butter. Drop by teaspoonfuls on greased cookie sheets. Bake for 10 minutes in a 350°F. oven. Remove from pan while warm. Makes 18.

PIES

CHOCOLATE CHIFFON PIE

1 envelope gelatin
¼ cup cold water
6 level tablespoons cocoa or 2 ounces chocolate
½ cup boiling water
4 EGGS, separated
1 cup cane, beet or fruit sugar
¼ teaspoon salt
1 teaspoon vanilla
Springform Pie Crust*
Whipped CREAM

Mix cocoa or chocolate and boiling water until smooth. Add gelatin to chocolate mixture, stirring thoroughly. Add egg yolks, slightly beaten, ½ cup of the sugar, salt and vanilla. Beat egg whites until stiff. Cook chocolate mixture and when it begins to thicken, fold in the egg whites and remaining ½ cup sugar. Pour into springform crust and chill. Just before serving, spread with a thin layer of whipped cream. Serves 6 to 8.

*See Springform Pie Crust recipe in Part 15.

RUM PIE

6 EGG yolks
1 cup corn-free sugar
2 envelopes gelatin
½ cup cold water
½ cup dark rum
2 cups heavy CREAM
Pie crust*
Semisweet chocolate

Beat egg yolks until light and lemon colored. Beat in sugar until thoroughly blended. Soak gelatin in cold water in small saucepan. Place over low heat and bring just to boil, stirring to dissolve gelatin. Remove from heat and pour over sugar-egg mixture, stirring constantly. Stir in rum. Whip cream until stiff. Fold into egg mixture and chill until it begins to set. Turn into crust and chill until firm. Just before serving sprinkle top of pie generously with shaved chocolate. Serves 8 to 10.

*See Springform Pie Crust recipe in Part 15.

PART 5

No Corn, No Egg, No Milk

BREADS

SWEDISH RYE BREAD

3 tablespoons Crisco
2 tablespoons cane, beet or fruit sugar
2 teaspoons salt
4 cups boiling water
1 cake yeast
3 cups rye FLOUR
1 cup wheat FLOUR

In evening, add Crisco, sugar and salt to boiling water. Cool. Add yeast, mixed with a little tepid water, to sugar, rye flour and flour mixture. Allow to rise. In the morning add more rye flour, a little at a time, to make a stiff dough. Let rise and knead again. Grease pie pans with Crisco. Bake in a 400°F. oven for ½ hour. Remove from oven and brush crust with a little melted Crisco. Makes 4 loaves.

BAKING POWDER BISCUITS

2 cups corn-free flour
4 teaspoons corn-free baking powder
1 teaspoon salt
2 tablespoons chicken fat
¾ to 1 cup water

Sift dry ingredients together. Rub the fat and flour together. Pour water gradually into mixture until soft enough to handle easily. Put on floured board and roll out ½ inch thick. Cut into round biscuits and bake at 425°F. to 450°F. in preheated oven for 15 minutes, or more. Makes 8 to 12, depending on size.

RICE FLOUR BISCUITS

- **1 cup rice FLOUR**
- **¼ teaspoon salt**
- **1 tablespoon corn-free baking powder**
- **2 tablespoons vegetable oil**
- **½ cup Sobee liquid**
- **½ cup water**
- **Cottonseed oil**

Combine flour, salt and baking powder in a large bowl. Add oil. Stir in Sobee liquid and water and mix well. Turn dough out on lightly floured board and knead lightly 10 times. Pat into biscuits. Bake in baking pan greased with cottonseed oil on rack slightly above center of a preheated 400°F. oven for 15 to 20 minutes. Bake until light brown. Makes 8 to 12.

POULTRY STUFFINGS

BREAD SUBSTITUTE STUFFING

- **1 cup matzo meal**
- **3 tablespoons fat, melted**
- **½ cup stewed tomatoes**
- **¼ teaspoon pepper or paprika**
- **1 tablespoon chopped onion (or bowl rubbed with garlic)**
- **¾ teaspoon salt**
- **⅛ teaspoon sage (optional)**

Brown matzo meal lightly in fat. Add all other ingredients, blending into a smooth stuffing. Use for a small chicken.

Note: Quantity can be doubled.

CHESTNUT STUFFING

3 cups shelled chestnuts
½ cup safflower oil
1 cup matzo meal
¼ cup cold water
1 teaspoon pepper or paprika (optional)

Blanch chestnuts and boil until soft in salted water. Drain. Add oil with matzo meal and cold water. Season with pepper or paprika. Brown matzo meal lightly in chicken fat. Mash chestnuts with fork and combine with meal, water and seasoning. Use for stuffing turkey.

SALAD DRESSING

SOY MAYONNAISE

1 cup water
½ cup Soyalac powder
½ teaspoon salt
½ teaspoon paprika
½ teaspoon Accent
1 cup corn-free oil
Juice of 1 lemon

Combine water, Soyalac, salt and seasoning in a blender container. Add oil gradually and lemon juice last. Also may be seasoned with onion or garlic. (You may use ¾ cup Soyalac liquid concentrate instead of ½ cup Soyalac powder and 1 cup water.)

When using an electric mixer, or a bowl and egg beater, use ½ cup water instead of 1 cup and increase oil to 1¼ cups. Beat together the water, Soyalac and seasonings. Add the oil slowly while beating. Then add the lemon juice. Makes approximately 3 cups.

Note: Keep mayonnaise in refrigerator. If it separates slightly, whip with a fork until smooth again.

SAUCES

WHITE SAUCE MADE WITH GOAT'S MILK

1 tablespoon chicken fat
1 tablespoon corn-free flour
½ cup goat's MILK*
½ cup cold water
Salt

Melt chicken fat, add flour and blend. Add goat's milk, which has been mixed with cold water. Allow to thicken. Season with a little salt. Makes about 1 cup.

*Goat's milk is used here as a substitute for cow's milk but does contain the same casein fraction as cow's milk.

BEVERAGES

SOYALAC FIG DRINK

½ cup Soyalac
¼ cup water
¼ cup Loma Linda fig juice (or Loma Linda prune juice)

Mix thoroughly and serve hot or cold. This makes a thick beverage, that may be thinned with ¼ cup water, if desired. Makes 1 cup.

CREAMY SOBEE LIQUID

1 cup Sobee liquid
½ cup water

Mix well and chill. Makes 1½ cups.

PART 6

No Corn, No Egg, No Wheat

BREADS

BREAD WITH POTATO AND RYE FLOUR

1 cup hot potato water
½ teaspoon cane, beet or fruit sugar
½ cake corn-free yeast (½ ounce)
2½ cups rye FLOUR
¼ cup potato flour
½ cup riced potatoes
1 teaspoon salt
1 teaspoon caraway seeds (optional)

Pour potato water or plain water into a mixing bowl. When lukewarm, add sugar and yeast dissolved in ⅛ cup tepid liquid. Stir in the remaining ingredients. Knead until smooth. Let rise in warm place until doubled in bulk. Put on board floured with potato flour. Form into loaves, place in greased pans and let rise again until doubled in bulk. Brush tops with water. Bake in 450°F. oven for 1 hour. Increase oven temperature to 500°F. first 20 minutes. Keep oven even 20 minutes; decrease to 400°F. last 20 minutes. Makes 2 loaves.

RYE BREAD

1 tablespoon fat
1 tablespoon cane, beet or fruit sugar
¾ teaspoon salt
½ cup boiling water
½ cup MILK
¼ yeast cake
1½ cups rye FLOUR

Add fat, sugar and salt to water and milk. When tepid, add yeast, which has been dissolved in ⅛ cup tepid water. Add half of the flour. Mix and let rise. When light, add remaining flour to make dough stiff enough to knead. When thoroughly kneaded, let rise again. Put in greased loaf pan. Cover and allow to rise once more. Bake at 400°F. for 1 hour. Makes 1 small loaf.

RICE SHEET BREAD

1 cup Cellu soybean flour
¾ cup Cellu rice flour
4 teaspoons Cellu baking powder
½ teaspoon salt
3 tablespoons cane, beet or fruit sugar
¼ cup corn-free fat, melted
1 cup plus 2 tablespoons cold water

Combine ingredients in order listed. This makes a medium thin batter. Pour batter (which should not exceed a ¼-inch thickness) into an 8x8-inch baking pan greased with corn-free fat. Bake at 400°F. for about 1 hour. Serves 6 to 8.

RYE MUFFINS

1 cup sifted rye FLOUR
2 teaspooons corn-free baking powder
¼ to ½ teaspoon salt
¼ cup Mull-Soy
¼ cup water
2 tablespoons corn-free margarine, melted
2 tablespoons molasses

Blend together rye flour, baking powder and salt and sift. Combine Mull-Soy, water, margarine and molasses. Pour Mull-Soy mixture all at once into dry ingredients, stirring until dry ingredients are dampened. Turn batter into well-greased 2-inch muffin cups, filling cups two-thirds full. Bake in a 400°F. oven for about 25 to 30 minutes, or until tops are browned. Makes 6 medium-sized muffins.

OAT BISCUITS

2 tablespoons oat flour
2 tablespoons soy fluff flour
1 teaspoon corn-free baking powder
¼ teaspoon salt
1 tablespoon corn-free shortening
2 tablespoons MILK

Mix dry ingredients and blend with shortening. Add milk. Roll into balls and pat flat. Bake on a greased baking tin in a preheated 450°F. oven for 20 to 30 minutes. Makes 8.

MEATS

MEAT-RICE PATTIES

½ pound ground beef
½ to ¾ teaspoon salt
¾ cup cooked rice
¼ cup Mull-Soy

Combine all the ingredients. Shape into patties, using ¼ cup of the mixture for each patty. Place on broiler pan, 3 inches from heat, and cook until browned. Turn and heat until browned on other side. Serve hot. Makes 6 patties.

SWISS STEAK

1 teaspoon salt
½ teaspoon pepper
½ cup potato flour
2½ pounds round steak
2 tablespoons chicken fat
½ chopped onion
½ green pepper, seeded and chopped fine
1½ cups water
½ cup catsup

Add salt and pepper to flour. Pound into meat. Brown in skillet with fat. Add onion, green pepper, water and catsup. Cover tightly and simmer slowly until tender, about 2 hours. You may also cook in oven at about 350°F. if desired. Serves 4 to 6.

POULTRY

POULTRY STUFFING

2 bouillon cubes
3 cups hot water
1½ teaspoons sage
2 teaspoons salt
¼ teaspoon pepper
2 quarts dark bread crumbs (made of rolled Swedish rye bread)
1½ to 2 onions, chopped
3 stalks celery, chopped
2 teaspoons dried parsley

Mix bouillon cubes into hot water. Stir seasonings into crumbs, then stir in other ingredients. Makes about 8 cups.

VEGETABLES

MASHED POTATOES

4 medium-sized potatoes
2 teaspoons soy margarine
1 teaspoon salt
Dash of pepper
2 cups Sobee liquid
2 cups water
Dash of paprika (optional)

Boil potatoes in covered pan for about 20 minutes until tender, then drain and mash well. Add margarine, salt, pepper mixing well. Heat Sobee liquid and water, mixed half and half. Beat all together until potatoes are light and fluffy. Add a dash of paprika before serving. Serves 4.

CANDY

PRALINES

2 cups powdered confectioners' cane, beet or fruit sugar
½ cup CREAM
1 cup maple syrup
2 cups whole pecans

Boil sugar, cream and maple syrup together until mixture forms a soft ball when tested in cold water. Beat until smooth and creamy. Cook 2 minutes at medium heat. Stir in nuts and drop from teaspoon in small lumps on waxed paper.

COOKIES

COCONUT MACAROONS

3 tablespoons Mull-Soy
2 tablespoons cane, beet or fruit sugar
¼ to ½ teaspoon salt
½ teaspoon vanilla
1 cup (¼-pound can) moist, sweetened coconut

Combine Mull-Soy, sugar, salt and vanilla. Stir in coconut. Drop by teaspoonfuls, about 1 inch apart, onto a greased cookie sheet. Bake at 350°F. until lightly browned, about 8 minutes. Makes about 12.

OATMEAL COOKIES

2 cups ground oatmeal
¾ cup BUTTER
¾ teaspoon vanilla
6 tablespoons confectioners' cane, beet or fruit sugar

Mix ingredients and drop in small cakes on a buttered cookie sheet. Bake in a 350°F. oven until brown (15 to 20 minutes). Place hot pan on wet cloth to remove cookies easily. Makes about 1½ to 2 dozen.

PINEAPPLE DROP COOKIES

½ cup corn-free shortening
½ cup corn-free brown sugar
½ cup corn-free white sugar
½ cup drained, crushed pineapple
1 cup barley flour
1 cup potato starch
¼ teaspoon salt
¼ teaspoon baking soda
1 tablespoon corn-free baking powder
½ cup chopped nuts

Cream shortening and sugars, then add pineapple. Combine dry ingredients and add to mixture. When well mixed, add nuts. Drop onto a well-greased cookie sheet and bake at 425°F. for about 12 minutes. Remove to rack to cool. Makes about 2 dozen.

ICEBOX COOKIES

- **½ cup corn-free shortening**
- **⅓ cup corn-free brown sugar**
- **⅓ cup corn-free white sugar**
- **1 teaspoon vanilla**
- **1 teaspoon corn-free baking powder**
- **⅓ cup Cellu rye flour**
- **⅛ teaspoon baking soda**
- **4 teaspoons warm water**
- **⅓ cup chopped pecans**

Cream shortening and sugars. Add vanilla, baking powder, flour and soda, moistened with water. Stir until smooth. Add pecans and form into roll. Chill and slice. Bake in a preheated 350°F. oven for 12 to 15 minutes. Makes about 1½ dozen.

PIE CRUST

RYE CRACKER CRUST

- **1½ cups crushed rye crackers**
- **⅓ cup confectioners' sugar, cane, beet or fruit**
- **½ cup BUTTER (or chicken fat, or other corn-free fat)**

Pat mixture on pie plate. Refrigerate for several hours. Fill with favorite fruit filling and chill. Makes 1 large pie crust.

PART 7

No Corn, No Milk, No Wheat

BREADS

RYE BREAD
(Icebox)

- **¼ cup chicken fat or corn-free vegetable oil**
- **¼ cup cane, beet, or fruit sugar**
- **¼ teaspoon salt**
- **¼ cup boiling water**
- **1 EGG, beaten**
- **½ cake yeast**
- **¼ cup cold water**
- **1½ cups rye FLOUR**
- **1 cup rice FLOUR**

Cream fat, sugar and salt. Stir in boiling water. Add egg and yeast, which has been dissolved in the cold water. Sift flours together and add. Refrigerate, covered, for at least 8 hours. Remove and shape dough into bread or rolls. Keep in greased pans for at least 4 hours at 80°F. Bake in a preheated 325°F. oven, 30 minutes for loaf, 25 minutes or more for rolls. Makes one loaf or 1 dozen large rolls.

GLUTEN-FREE RICE BREAD

2 cups rice FLOUR
¼ cup potato starch
½ cup milk substitute (solid)
1½ to 2 tablespoons cane, beet or fruit sugar
1 tablespoon corn-free baking powder
1 teaspoon salt
2 EGGS
⅓ cup corn-free cooking oil
⅞ cup water

Combine dry ingredients. Beat eggs in small bowl and while beating, add oil. Continue to beat vigorously until thick and smooth. Add water and beat until mixed. Add to dry ingredients and stir lightly until blended (do not overmix). Pour into a 4x8-inch loaf pan greased with corn-free oil. Let stand about 4 minutes before placing in oven. Bake in a preheated 350°F. oven for 1 hour. Remove from pan and cool on wire rack. Makes approximately 16 to 18 ½-inch slices.

OAT MUFFINS

1 tablespoon cane, beet or fruit sugar
½ teaspoon salt
1 tablespoon corn-free margarine
1 EGG
½ cup oat flour
½ cup soy fluff flour
2 teaspoons corn-free baking powder
¾ cup water

Mix sugar, salt and margarine. Blend in beaten egg. Sift flours and baking powder. Add to sugar mixture, alternating with water. Batter should not be stiff—add more water if necessary. Grease muffin tins and fill halfway. Bake in a preheated 450°F. oven for about 30 minutes. Makes 1 dozen small muffins.

POTATO FLOUR MUFFINS

½ cup potato flour
1 tablespoon cane, beet or fruit sugar
4 EGGS
2 tablespoons water

Mix dry ingredients and sift. Beat eggs, add water and stir in dry ingredients. Turn into greased muffin tins. Bake at 450°F. for 20 to 30 minutes. Makes 6 to 8.

RICE MUFFINS

4 cups rice FLOUR
4 teaspoons corn-free baking powder
2 teaspoons salt
1 cup cane, beet or fruit sugar
2 EGGS
1½ cups water and 1½ cups Soyalac liquid, combined
2 tablespoons corn-free margarine, melted

Sift dry ingredients. Combine egg, water-Soyalac mixture and shortening. Add to the dry ingredients, stirring just enough to combine. Fill greased muffin pans about half full. Bake in a 400°F. oven for about 25 minutes. Makes 2 dozen.

BARLEY GRIDDLE CAKES

1 teaspoon soy margarine, melted
½ cup Soyalac concentrated liquid
½ cup water
1 EGG, beaten
1 cup barley flour
2 teaspoons corn-free baking powder
¼ teaspoon salt

Blend liquid ingredients, then combine dry ingredients. Pour liquid ingredients into the dry, stirring until mixture is smooth. Bake in small cakes on a preheated griddle until each cake is full of bubbles and the undersurface is brown. Turn and brown on other side. Serve hot. Makes six average-sized cakes.

YUMMY COCONUT PANCAKES

1¼ cups rice FLOUR
¼ teaspoon salt
1½ cups cane, beet or fruit sugar
4 EGGS
3 cups coconut milk
½ cup corn-free cooking oil

Sift flour, salt and sugar into a bowl. Beat in eggs and coconut milk until very smooth. Heat 2 teaspoons of oil in a skillet. Lightly brown pancakes on both sides. Roll up like a jelly roll. Repeat for each pancake. Keep warm until ready to serve. Makes about 2½ dozen.

DESSERTS

Cakes

CARROT CAKE

5 EGG yolks, beaten
1 cup cane, beet or fruit sugar
2 tablespooons potato flour
1 teaspoon allspice
1 teaspoon cinnamon
1 teaspoon vanilla
½ cup ground carrots
1 cup chopped nuts
Pinch salt
5 EGG whites, beaten

To the egg yolks add remaining ingredients, beaten egg whites last. Preheat oven to 400°F. and bake in two layers for 40 to 50 minutes. Serves 12 to 14.

RICE CAKES

4 EGG whites
⅓ cup cane, beet or fruit sugar
1 cup rice FLOUR
1 teaspoon vanilla
½ cup softened soy butter

Beat egg whites slightly. Add sugar and twice-sifted flour, stirring it in very lightly. Add vanilla and butter. Drop on a greased cookie sheet 2 to 3 inches apart. Use the back of a floured spoon to spread thin. Bake in a moderate oven at 325°F. to 350°F. for 10 minutes. They will be thin and crisp.

JELLY ROLL

Potato Flour Sponge Cake* cooked in a 10x15-inch pan. Spread with jelly and roll. Dust with powdered cane, beet or fruit sugar.

*SPONGE CAKE

4 tablespoons cane, beet or fruit sugar
4 EGG whites, stiffly beaten
4 EGG yolks
1 level teaspoon baking powder (corn-free)
5 tablespoons potato flour
Vanilla

Add sugar to egg whites. Add yolks and remaining ingredients. Transfer to oblong pan lined with greased waxed paper. Bake in a preheated 325°F. oven for 40 minutes. Serves 8 to 10.

CAROB ROLL

6 EGGS, separated
1 cup cane, beet or fruit sugar
1 cup carob
Mint jelly

Cream egg yolks and sugar together. Beat egg whites until stiff and add to yolks with the carob. Grease waxed paper with either chicken fat or some cottonseed product, on both sides. Bake in a preheated 275°F. oven for about 15 minutes. Cover with mint jelly and roll when cold. Put on flat platter and sprinkle with powdered sugar. Serves 4 to 6.

CAROB BROWNIES

2 EGGS
½ cup, less 4 tablespoons sifted rice or rye FLOUR
1 teaspoon vanilla
1¼ cups cane, beet or fruit sugar
½ cup chopped nuts
½ cup carob

Beat eggs slightly. Stir in remaining ingredients. Spread evenly in an 8x8x2-inch pan. Bake at 375°F. for 20 minutes. Makes about 2½ dozen.

NUT AND BUTTER CAKE

½ cup barley flour
½ cup rye FLOUR
½ cup potato flour
Pinch of salt
1 teaspoon corn-free baking powder
½ cup corn-free margarine
1 cup cane, beet or fruit sugar
2 EGGS, separated
6 tablespoons Soyamel
½ cup chopped nuts
1 teaspoon vanilla

Sift flours with salt and baking powder. Cream shortening and sugar then beat in egg yolks. Mix until creamy. Add the Soyamel and flour mixture alternately, beating well. Add nuts. Add vanilla. Stiffly beat whites and fold in. Pour into a greased pan and bake in a 350°F. oven for 25 to 30 minutes. Serves 8.

Cookies

ALMOND COOKIES

- **¾ cup almonds**
- **2 tablespoons cold water**
- **1 tablespoon vinegar**
- **5 EGGS, separated**
- **4 tablespoons corn-free fat, melted**
- **½ teaspoon corn-free baking powder**
- **Pinch of salt**

Blanch almonds. Bake until light brown, then put through a grater. Place in a strainer. Combine cold water and vinegar, pour over almonds and drain. Dry in oven. Grind again. Beat egg yolks until thick and lemon colored. Combine almonds with yolks, melted fat, baking powder and salt. Stiffly beat egg whites and fold in. Fill greased gem pans ⅔ full. Bake in 300°F. oven for 25 minutes. Makes 9 large cookies.

ALMOND PASTE FOR MACAROONS

- **2 EGG whites**
- **1¾ cups confectioners' cane, beet or fruit sugar**
- **1 teaspoon lemon juice**
- **½ pound shelled almonds**

Beat egg whites until foamy. Gradually add sugar and lemon juice. Blanch almonds, chop fine with knife, then grind in food chopper. Repeat several times. When fine enough add to egg and sugar mixture. It should be smooth and creamy. If too stiff, add lemon juice, drop by drop. Allow to stand 24 hours before using. (Prepared almond paste can be purchased.) Makes about 2½ cups.

DATE AND WALNUT DROPS

4 EGG whites
⅓ teaspoon cream of tartar
1½ cups cane, beet or fruit sugar
1 cup chopped walnuts
½ pound dates, cut in pieces
2 or 3 drops vanilla or almond extract

Beat egg whites until foamy. Add cream of tartar and beat stiff. Add 1¼ cups of the sugar and beat until mixture holds its shape. Fold in the remaining ¼ cup sugar. Add nuts and dates and vanilla or almond extract. Drop on buttered and floured cookie sheets, about the size of silver dollar, leaving 1 inch between. Bake in a preheated 250°F. oven for 30 to 50 minutes. Cakes should dry out rather than bake. Makes 2½ dozen, depending on size.

Puddings

APRICOT FLUFF

1 (16-ounce) can apricots
1 tablespoon lemon juice
2 EGG whites, stiffly beaten

Put apricots through ricer. Add lemon juice and egg whites. Put in freezer tray of refrigerator and allow to harden for 2½ to 3 hours. Makes 6 to 8.

BANANA WHIP

2 small bananas
4 tablespoons confectioners' cane, beet or fruit sugar
1 tablespoon lemon juice
2 EGG whites, stiffly beaten

Rice bananas and add sugar and lemon juice. Fold in egg whites. Freeze in refrigerator for 2½ to 3 hours. Makes about 1 cup.

CABINET PUDDING

1 dozen homemade macaroons
1 cup sherry
6 tablespoons cane, beet or fruit sugar
6 EGGS, separated
2 envelopes gelatin
¼ cup cold water
¼ cup hot water
1 cup crushed macaroons

Line a mold with macaroons. Heat sherry in the top of a double boiler. Combine sugar and egg yolks, then add to sherry. Thicken. Dissolve gelatin in cold water. Thin with hot water. Pour gelatin into sherry custard. When thoroughly dissolved, add crushed macaroons and cool slightly. Stiffly beat egg whites and fold in. Pour into 6 cup mold. Chill for 6 hours.

WINE CUSTARD

6 EGGS
6 tablespoons cane, beet or fruit sugar
6 tablespoons sweet sherry

Combine eggs, sugar and sherry in top of a double boiler. Beat until frothy. Cook over hot (but not boiling) water, beating mixture until it begins to bubble. Remove top of boiler at once and place in cool water. Continue beating until thickened. Pour into sherbet glasses. May be served warm or cold. Serves 4 to 6.

PART 8

No Corn, No Egg, No Milk, No Wheat

BREADS

RYE BREAD

1 cake yeast, crumbled
½ cup lukewarm water
½ cup Sobee liquid
2 tablespoons corn-free vegetable oil
4 teaspoons cane, beet or fruit sugar
1 teaspoon salt
3 cups sifted rye FLOUR

Dissolve yeast in ¼ cup of the lukewarm water. Mix together Sobee, vegetable oil, sugar, salt and the remaining ¼ cup water. Add 1 cup sifted flour and beat until smooth. Stir in dissolved yeast, beating well. Work in remaining 2 cups flour gradually.

Turn out onto a floured board and kneed until dough is smooth. Dough may be a little moist but should be workable if handled lightly. Put into a bowl greased with corn-free fat and turn dough once to bring greased side up. Cover with damp cloth and let stand in warm place (80°F. to 85°F.) until dough is doubled in bulk. (To tell when dough has doubled, press deeply with fingers, then lift fingers. If holes do not close, dough has doubled and is ready to rework.) Turn out on board and work again for about 5 minutes. Shape dough into smooth loaf and place in greased pan. Grease top of loaf with corn-free vegetable shortening, cover and let rise until double in bulk. Bake in a

375°F. oven for about 45 minutes, or until well browned. Makes 1 loaf.

YEAST RAISED RICE BREAD

2½ cups warm water (100°F.)
1 package yeast, active dry or compressed
¼ cup corn-free sugar
¼ cup corn-free vegetable oil
1 (24-ounce) package Jolly Joan Rice Mix

Pour water into a bowl and dissolve yeast. Stir in sugar and oil. Slowly add rice mix. Stir until dough is smooth, about 3 to 5 minutes. Cover bowl with damp cloth and let rise in warm place (about 80°F.) for 30 minutes. Stir batter again with a spoon for 5 minutes. Pour dough into two 8x4x2-inch bread pans. Cover pans with damp cloth and let rise in warm place (about 80°F.) for 45 minutes. Bake in a preheated 350°F. oven for 50 minutes, or until brown. Turn loaves out on wire racks to cool. Makes 2 loaves.

BISCUITS

1 cup rice FLOUR
¼ teaspoon salt
1 tablespoon corn-free baking powder
2 tablespoons corn-free vegetable oil
½ cup Sobee liquid
½ cup water

Combine the first three ingredients in large bowl, then add oil. Mix Sobee and water, then add to dry ingredients. Turn dough out on lightly floured board and knead lightly 10 times. Pat into biscuits. Place in a baking pan which has been greased with corn-free fat. Bake at 400°F. for about 18 to 20 minutes or until brown (have your rack slightly above center of oven). Makes 8 large or 12 small biscuits.

SOYALAC RYE MUFFINS

¼ cup Soyalac (concentrated liquid)
¼ cup water
2 tablespoons corn-free oil
2 tablespoons honey, molasses, or beet, cane or fruit sugar
1 cup rye FLOUR
2 teaspoons corn-free baking powder
¼ teaspoon salt

Combine all liquid ingredients. Sift rye flour, baking powder and salt together and add to liquid ingredients. Mix thoroughly. Place batter in muffin tins, filling about two-thirds full. Bake in a 400°F. oven for 25 to 30 minutes, or until nicely browned. Makes 8 large or 12 small muffins.

SOYALAC WAFFLES

1 cup Soyalac
1 cup FLOUR (any flour allowed)
1 tablespoon vegetable oil
½ teaspoon salt
1 tablespoon cane, beet or fruit sugar or brown sugar

Combine all the ingredients, mixing well. Bake in hot waffle iron until nicely brown. These waffles are raised by steam and take a few minutes longer than other types. You must use a heavy waffle iron for success with this recipe. Makes 2 or 3.

RICE PANCAKES

1 cup cooked rice
2 tablespoons minced scallions
2 tablespoons minced green pepper
2 tablespoons minced celery
2 tablespoons minced water chestnuts
2 teaspoons Jolly Joan Egg Replacer plus 2 tablespoons water*
¼ teaspoon salt
Pepper
2 tablespoons corn-free oil
Sauce Soy**

Combine rice, scallions, pepper, celery, water chestnuts, egg replacer and water, salt and pepper. Heat oil in skillet and add rice and egg mixture. Spread gently to cover bottom of pan. Cook over low heat until set. Loosen carefully with spatula and transfer to a hot serving plate. Serve with Sauce Soy. Serves 4.

*1 teaspoon Jolly Joan Egg Replacer plus 1 tablespoon water is equal to one egg.

**See under Sauces, Part 12.

Candy

FUDGE

¾ cup soy milk
1 cup El Molino carob powder
¼ cup soy margarine
2 cups dark brown cane, beet or fruit sugar
1 teaspoon vanilla
½ teaspoon lemon extract
Chopped nuts

Combine milk, carob powder and margarine. Cook, stirring, over medium heat until smooth and thick. Add sugar, stirring until sugar is thoroughly dissolved, but do not stir after mixture starts to boil. Cook to firm ball stage when tested in cold water. Cool without stirring to lukewarm, then add vanilla and lemon extract. Beat until thick. Add nuts, and pour into 8″x8″ pan which has been greased with corn-free oil. When cold, cut into squares. Makes 16 ½-inch pieces or 8 1-inch pieces.

SECTION II

EGG ALLERGY

INTRODUCTION

Wheat, milk and corn bother more people than eggs do, but an allergic reaction to eggs is often much more severe. A truly highly sensitive person may not even be able to shake hands with someone who has eaten eggs. An ever so slightly impure vaccine containing a minuscule amount of egg can render him incommunicative.

Eggs are a good source of protein; an average egg contains about the same amount of protein as 8 ounces of whole milk and ⅓ as much as ¼ pound of lean cooked beef.

Dried eggs, powdered eggs, buried Chinese eggs, turkey eggs are EGGS! All eggs are the same although the birds from which they come are not.

Ener-G Cereal Inc. makes Jolly Joan Egg Replacer, which is egg, milk and wheat free but does contain corn. One teaspoon of the replacer mixed with one tablespoon of water will substitute for one egg in most recipes, although it is not nutritionally the same.

Egg is found in the following:

Baked eggs
Baking powders*
Batters for French frying
Bavarian cream
Boiled dressings
Bouillons
Breads
Breaded foods
Cakes
Cake flours

Candies, except hard
Chicken
Coffee, if cleared with egg
Consommés
Coddled eggs
Cookies*
Creamed eggs
Creamed pies
Croquettes
Custards
Deviled eggs
Dessert powders
Doughnuts
Dried eggs
Dried eggs in prepared foods
Dumplings
Egg albumin
Escalloped eggs
Fried eggs
Fritters
Frostings
French toast
Griddle cakes
Glazed rolls
Hard-cooked eggs
Hamburger mix
Hollandaise sauce
Ices
Ice Cream
Icings
Laxative, Agarol
Macaroons
Malted cocoa drinks
Macaroni
Meat loaf
Meat jellies
Marshmallows
Meat molds
Meringues
Noodles*
Omelets
Ovaltine
Ovomalt
Pastes
Pancakes
Pancake flour
Patties
Poached eggs
Puddings
Pretzels
Salad dressings
Sauces
Sausages
Sherbets
Shirred eggs
Soft-cooked eggs
Soufflés
Soups
Spaghetti*
Spanish creams
Tartar sauce
Timbales
Waffles
Waffle mixes
Whips
Wines (many wines are cleared with egg whites)

You must determine if egg is used in your own brands of pastries, puddings and ice creams. Dried or powdered eggs are often overlooked. Also some individuals who are allergic to eggs may be allergic to chicken, too, and they should consider this prior to using Chicken recipes.

*Some brands are free of egg.

PART 9

No Egg

BREADS

CHEESE BISCUITS

1½ cups FLOUR
¼ teaspoon salt
2 teaspoons baking powder
1 teaspoon shortening
6 tablespoons grated CHEESE
⅝ cup MILK

Sift together dry ingredients. Add shortening and cheese. Add just enough milk to hold dough together. Roll on floured board to a ½-inch thickness. Cut with small cutter. Bake in a 450°F. oven for 15 minutes. Makes 12 large or 16 small biscuits.

RICE AND RYE FLOUR BREAD (See Part 12)

RYE BREAD (See Part 12)

SOUTHERN CORN PONE (See Part 12)

CROUTONS (See Part 12)

CINNAMON TOAST (See Part 12)

RICE MUFFINS (See Part 12)

SOYALAC PANCAKES (See Part 12)

SOYALAC CORN STICKS (See Part 12)

RYE BAKING POWDER BREAD (See Part 11)

EGGLESS NUT BREAD (See Part 11)

BARLEY BREAD (See Part 11)

CORNBREAD (See Part 11)

RYE AND CORNMEAL MUFFINS (See Part 11)

CORNMEAL CAKES (See Part 11)

PANCAKES (See Part 11)

RYE POTATO BREAD

¼ cup mashed potatoes
1½ tablespoons cane, beet or fruit sugar
½ teaspoon salt
½ tablespoon fat
¼ cup potato water
½ yeast cake
1 cup rye FLOUR
½ cup potato flour

Mix potato, sugar, salt and fat until smooth. Heat potato water to lukewarm and dissolve yeast. Add to potato mixture. Combine flours and sift into batter. Set batter aside in warm place until it doubles in bulk, about 4 hours. Knead again. Form into a loaf. Place in a greased pan and let rise. Preheat oven to 450°F.; bake, increasing heat to 500°F. in 20 minutes, keeping even at 500°F. for 20 minutes, decreasing to 350°F. for 20 minutes. Makes 1 small loaf.

RAISIN BREAD

½ cup molasses
1½ cups hot water
¼ cup chopped, seeded raisins
⅓ cup brown sugar
1½ cups soybean FLOUR
1 teaspoon salt
1½ cups CORNSTARCH or rice FLOUR
½ teaspoon baking soda
1 tablespoon baking powder
1 tablespoon CORN OIL or olive oil

Combine molasses and ¾ cup of the hot water. Pour remaining ¾ cup water over raisins and add to molasses. Add remaining ingredients in order, oil last. Bake in well-greased bread pan in a 350°F. oven for about 1½ hours. Makes 1 or 2 loaves.

SOYALAC CORN BREAD

1 cup Soyalac
1 cup water
¼ cup oil
3 tablespoons honey, molasses or sugar
2 cups yellow CORNMEAL
1½ teaspoons salt
1 tablespoon baking powder

Combine liquids and blend dry ingredients. Pour liquids into the cornmeal mixture, stirring only until dry ingredients are dampened. Put batter into an oiled 8x8x2-inch pan, spreading evenly with a spoon. Bake at 450°F. for about 20 minutes, or until center top is firm when lightly touched. Allow to cool for 5 minutes before cutting into 2-inch squares and removing from pan. Serve hot or cold. Serves 4.

SWEET POTATO BISCUITS

2 large sweet potatoes, boiled
1 cup cane, beet or fruit sugar
2 teaspoons BUTTER or CORN OIL
4 cups FLOUR
Pinch of salt
1 tablespoon baking powder
MILK

Mash potatoes and add sugar and butter. Sift flour, salt and baking powder and add to potato mixture. Make into a soft dough with milk. Roll out and cut into biscuit shapes. Bake in a preheated 450°F. oven for about 20 minutes. Makes about 2 dozen.

CORN PONE

¼ cup CORNMEAL
⅓ teaspoon salt
½ cup boiling water

After sifting dry ingredients, scald with water. Grease griddle or frying pan. Make into 1 large or 4 small cakes.

WAFFLES

1 cup FLOUR
½ teaspoon baking powder
½ teaspoon salt
¾ cup BUTTERMILK
¼ teaspoon baking soda
1½ teaspoons shortening, melted
½ teaspoon sugar

Sift together flour, baking powder and salt. Combine with buttermilk. Add soda, dissolved in a little water. Add shortening and sugar, mixing well. Heat iron 10 minutes before needed. Cook each waffle 4 minutes. Makes 2 or 3.

DUMPLINGS

1 cup FLOUR
½ teaspoon salt
1 tablespoon baking powder
6 tablespoons MILK

Sift dry ingredients together. Mix to a soft dough with the milk. Drop by spoonfuls into hot stew or broth and steam, covered, for 20 minutes. Makes 6.

CEREALS

CORNMEAL MUSH (See Part 12)

GRITS (See Part 12)

OATMEAL (See Part 12)

MEATS

MEAT LOAF

6 ounces ground beef
2 teaspoons chopped onion
4 tablespoons oatmeal
4 tablespoons tomato juice
4 to 6 measure Nutramigen powder
Salt, pepper, garlic to taste
Dash of catsup

Combine all ingredients, except catsup, mixing well. Place in loaf pan greased with corn-free oil. Top with catsup. Bake in a 350°F. oven for about 40 minutes, or until done. Serves 2.

HAMBURGER PATTIE

6 ounces ground beef
2 teaspoons chopped onion
Salt and pepper to taste
4 measures Nutramigen powder

Combine all ingredients and pat into desired shape. Brown well on each side in corn-free vegetable oil. Turn often until done. Serves 2.

Poultry

CHICKEN AND BROCCOLI DIVINE

2 chickens cut up
2 bunches broccoli
3 tablespoons soy BUTTER
¼ cup light CREAM
Salt (1⅛ tablespoons)
Cayenne pepper
Nutmeg
1¼ sticks corn-free margarine
1 small onion, chopped fine
6 tablespoons rice FLOUR
3 cups MILK
¼ cup grated American CHEESE
½ cup Parmesan CHEESE

Cut the broccoli lengthwise in equal-size pieces. Remove hard stems and stand upright in a tall pot. Add salted, boiling water. Cover and boil for 8 to 10 minutes or until tender. Drain and put through sieve. Stir in 3 tablespoons soy butter, then the cream. Add salt, pepper and nutmeg to taste. Set aside while you make the Cheese sauce.

CHEESE SAUCE: melt 7 tablespoons of margarine over a very low flame in deep, heavy skillet. Then add the minced onion. Sauté for a couple of minutes snd slowly stir in flour, then gradually add the milk, still stirring. When the mixture is smooth and thickened, stir in all the American cheese and half the Parmesan. Season to taste with salt, pepper and nutmeg. Combine all but one cup of sauce with the chicken. Pour into a 9x13x2-inch greased oven-to-table dish, then use remaining sauce on top. Sprinkle remaining Parmesan cheese, dot with margarine and place under broiler. After this is lightly browned keep warm by putting into oven at lowest setting. Heat broccoli and line edges of serving dish. Serves 5 to 6.

POULTRY (See Part 15)

FRIED CHICKEN

Frying chicken, cut up
Salt
Pepper (optional)
CORNFLAKES, crushed
Cooking fat or oil

Dissect chicken at joints; singe by holding over flame. Wash, season with salt, pepper and cornflakes. Heat cooking fat or oil very hot (when piece of bread dropped into fat browns in 1 minute). Heat chicken until a golden brown. Lower heat and brown on other side. Allow about 18 to 20 minutes. Serves 4.

Poultry Stuffing

OYSTER STUFFING

3 cups matzo meal (or cracker meal containing no milk)
½ cup melted chicken fat or vegetable oil
2½ teaspoons salt
½ teaspoon paprika or pepper (optional)
1 pint raw oysters, chopped, and liquor

Brown matzo meal lightly in fat. Season. Add oysters and liquor, blending all until smooth. Use as a chicken or turkey stuffing. Makes approximately 5 cups.

RICE STUFFING

¼ cup finely chopped crisp bacon
1 tablespoon chopped parsley
⅔ cup stewed tomatoes
2 cups cooked rice
1 tablespoon minced onion
½ teaspoon salt
⅛ teaspoon pepper (optional)

To bacon add all remaining ingredients in order. (Use as filling for breast of veal, also.) Makes approximately 3 cups.

POTATO STUFFING

2 teaspoons chopped onion (or garlic)
¼ cup melted chicken fat or bacon fat
1 cup matzo meal or CORN PONE (eggless, milkless)*
1 cup mashed potato (without milk or butter)
1¼ cups hot soup stock
¼ cup crisp, chopped bacon
⅛ teaspoon pepper or paprika
½ teaspoon salt

Brown onion in fat (if allergic to onion, rub pan with garlic before heating fat). Brown matzo crumbs lightly and add to mashed potato. Thin with soup stock. Blend until all is smooth, then add bacon and seasonings. Use to stuff poultry, green peppers, tomatoes or breast of veal. Makes 3½ to 3¾ cups.

*See recipe under Breads, this section.

HOECAKE STUFFING

2 tablespoons BUTTER
1 quart boiling water
2 cups CORNMEAL, scalded
2 teaspoons salt
3 stalks celery, chopped
1 pint water
1 chicken gizzard
1 chicken liver

Melt butter in skillet. Mix scalded cornmeal and salt. Spread in greased skillet to make a hoecake. Cover pan and cook on top of stove. Crumble bread after cooling. Stew celery in the 1 pint water until tender with gizzard and liver. Chop, then add celery water and season. Mix with hoecake. Thicken with cornmeal. Use as stuffing. Makes about 2 quarts.

VEGETABLES

CABBAGE AU GRATIN

½ large cabbage, cooked
¾ cup grated CHEESE
Salt and paprika
2 cups White Sauce (recipe follows)
½ cup cracker crumbs
3 tablespoons BUTTER, melted

Put a layer of cabbage, coarsely chopped, into a buttered baking dish. Sprinkle with cheese, salt and paprika as needed. Cover with a layer of white sauce. Repeat layers until all ingredients have been used, ending with a layer of white sauce. Cover with cracker crumbs mixed with butter. Keep in oven only long enough to make very hot and crumbs are brown. Serves 4.

WHITE SAUCE

2 tablespoons BUTTER
2 tablespoons FLOUR
1 cup hot MILK
½ teaspoon salt
⅙ teaspoon pepper

Melt butter in a saucepan. Remove from heat and mix flour in. Cook until it bubbles, then add ⅔ of the hot milk at once, and the rest gradually. Boil, stirring constantly, until the mixture thickens. Season (pepper is optional) and serve hot.

CORN FRITTERS

1 (17-ounce) can crushed CORN
1 tablespoon shortening, melted
2 teaspoons salt
¼ teaspoon white pepper
1 cup FLOUR
1 teaspoon baking powder
3 tablespoons MILK

Put corn into a bowl. Add shortening, salt, pepper, flour, baking powder and milk. Mix well. Drop by spoonfuls on a greased griddle. Fry brown on both sides. Makes 12.

SALADS

FRUIT-CHEESE SALAD

1 (16-ounce or 28-ounce) Queen Anne white cherries
1 (20-ounce) can crushed pineapple
½ package lime Jell-O (Use other flavors for other colors)
½ pound marshmallow tidbits
½ pound slivered toasted almonds
Dash of cayenne pepper
½ pound grated CHEESE
Pinch of salt
1 cup CREAM, whipped
1 cup eggless mayonnaise*

Pit and drain cherries. Drain pineapple and heat juice. Dissolve Jell-O in juice, then add marshmallows to melt. Allow to cool slightly and add the remaining ingredients except cream and mayonnaise, mixing well. Add cream. Refrigerate until it begins to set, then whip in mayonnaise. Pour into 12 to 16-cup mold and chill. Serves 8 to 10.

*See recipe under Salad Dressings, this section.

CRANBERRY RING

1½ cups hot water
1 package strawberry Jell-O
1 can cranberry sauce
Chopped pecans or almonds
Egg-free mayonnaise*
Lettuce

Pour water over Jell-O. Mix in cranberry sauce and nuts. Pour entire mixture into a 6-cup mold. When set serve with eggless mayonnaise on lettuce. Serves 6.

*See recipe under Salad Dressings, this section.

DELICIOUS JELLO SALAD

¾ cup tomato soup
1 (8-ounce) or 3 (3-ounce) packages CREAM CHEESE
2 packages lemon Jell-O
1 cup hot water
1 cup cold water
1 cup egg-free mayonnaise*
1 cup finely diced celery
1 cup finely diced cucumber
1 cup diced green stuffed olives
1 small onion, diced fine

Heat soup in the top of a double boiler. When hot add cream cheese and beat until smooth. Dissolve Jell-O in hot water, then add the cold water. Combine with the tomato mixture. When cool add mayonnaise and vegetables. Rub 10- to 12-cup mold with egg-free mayonnaise before pouring in salad. Refrigerate. When set turn out on lettuce. Serves 12.

*See recipe under Salad Dressings, this section.

BEET SALAD

- 1 (16-ounce) can diced beets
- 1 package lemon Jell-O
- ½ cup finely diced celery
- ⅕ cup vinegar
- 1 tablespoon horseradish
- 1 tablespoon chopped onion
- ⅓ teaspoon salt
- ⅛ teaspoon pepper
- Lettuce
- Egg-free mayonnaise*

Drain beets and heat the beet juice. Dissolve lemon Jell-O in hot juice. Add other ingredients in order. Pour into a 6-cup mold and chill. Serve with egg-free mayonnaise on lettuce. Serves 6 to 8.

*See recipe under Salad Dressings, this section.

CRANBERRY MOLD

- 2 cups cranberries
- 1½ cups water
- 1 cup sugar
- 1 package cherry Jell-O
- 1 cup crushed pineapple
- Juice of pineapple
- 1 tart apple, chopped fine
- ½ cup chopped nuts

Simmer cranberries in water for 10 minutes. Add sugar and stir. Add Jell-O and stir. Remove from heat and when cool add pineapple, a little juice, apple and nuts. Pour into a mold. Refrigerate. When firm serve on lettuce. Serves 4 to 6.

Salad Dressings

EGGLESS MAYONNAISE

- ½ teaspoon salt
- ½ teaspoon dry mustard
- Few grains of cayenne pepper
- ¼ teaspoon sugar
- 3 tablespoons evaporated MILK
- ¾ cup peanut oil (or salad or olive oil)
- 2 tablespoons vinegar or lemon juice

Mix first four ingredients together. Add milk and blend thoroughly. Gradually beat in oil. Add vinegar or lemon juice, beating until mixture is smooth. Makes about 1 cup.

*EGG-FREE MAYONNAISE

½ teaspoon salt
½ teaspoon dry mustard
¼ teaspoon paprika
½ teaspoon cane, beet or fruit sugar
Few grains of cayenne pepper
3 tablespoons evaporated MILK
¾ cup corn-free salad oil
2 tablespoons vinegar or lemon juice

Mix together dry ingredients and blend all with milk. Gradually beat in salad oil. Add vinegar or lemon juice and beat until smooth. Makes 1 cup.

OLIVE DRESSING

1 cup egg-free mayonnaise*
½ cup minced pimentos

Combine ingredients.

*See recipe under Salad Dressings, this section.

PIMIENTO DRESSING

½ cup finely cut pimiento CHEESE
1 cup egg-free mayonnaise*

Combine all ingredients. Makes 1 cup.

*See recipe under Salad Dressings, this section.

SOY MAYONNAISE (See recipe Part 5)

POTATO MAYONNAISE

1 very small baked potato
1 teaspoon mustard (optional)
1 teaspoon salt
1 teaspoon confectioners' sugar
2 tablespoons vinegar or lemon juice
¾ cup salad oil

Remove potato from skin and mash. Add mustard, salt and sugar. Add I tablespoon vinegar or lemon juice and rub mixture through fine sieve. Add oil and remaining vinegar or lemon slowly, beating well. Makes about 1 cup.

CREAM CHEESE DRESSING

1 (3-ounce) package CREAM CHEESE
1 cup eggless mayonnaise*

Whip cream cheese until fluffy. Fold into mayonnaise. Makes 1¼ cups.

*See recipe under Salad Dressings, this section.

DESSERTS

Cakes

STRAWBERRY SHORTCAKE

2 cups FLOUR
1 tablespoon baking powder
1 tablespoon sugar
½ teaspoon salt
4 tablespoons shortening
½ cup water
1 quart strawberries*
Whipped CREAM, sweetened

Sift together flour, baking powder, sugar and salt. Add shortening and mix thoroughly with a steel fork. Add water to make a soft dough. Roll out on floured board about ½ inch thick. Cut with large biscuit cutter dipped in flour, or half fill 6 large greased muffin rings that have been placed on a baking pan. Bake at 475°F. for 10 to 12 minutes. Split while hot, butter and fill with crushed sweetened berries. Put on tops and cover with strawberries and sweetened whipped cream. Serves 6.

*Any other fruit may be substituted for strawberries.

CHOCOLATE CAKE SQUARES

2 cups brown sugar
2 tablespoons BUTTER
8 tablespoons cocoa or carob
3 cups FLOUR
2 teaspoons baking soda
1½ cups MILK
½ teaspoon vanilla
Boiled Chocolate Icing* or Creamy Carob Icing*

Cream sugar, butter and cocoa. Sift together flour and baking soda, then stir in milk and vanilla. Preheat oven at 450°F. for 10 minutes. Bake in sheet tins for 20 minutes. Cut into squares. Makes 2 to 2½ dozen.

*See recipes for Boiled Chocolate Icing and Creamy Carob Icing in Part 15.

APPLESAUCE CAKE

1 level teaspoon baking soda
1½ cups hot applesauce
½ cup BUTTER
1 cup cane, beet or fruit sugar
2 cups corn-free flour
1½ cups raisins
1 teaspoon ground cloves
2 teaspoons cinnamon
1 cup chopped nuts

Stir soda into hot applesauce. Add the remaining ingredients. Bake in a 8x8-inch greased pan in a preheated oven at 400°F. for 45 to 50 minutes. Serves 6 to 8.

WHITE CAKE WITH CHOCOLATE ICING

- **1 cup cane, beet or fruit sugar**
- **⅓ cup BUTTER**
- **2 cups corn-free flour**
- **½ teaspoon salt**
- **½ teaspoon baking powder**
- **½ teaspoon baking soda**
- **1½ cups sour MILK**
- **Boiled Chocolate Icing***

Cream sugar and butter together. Sift flour, salt and baking powder. Combine baking soda and sour milk and add to the creamed mixture. Add dry ingredients. Grease two 9″ layer cake tins. Bake in a preheated 350°F. oven for 30 minutes. Frost with Boiled Chocolate Icing. Serves 8 to 10.

*See recipe under Icings in Part 15.

CAKE À LA DOBBS

- **½ cup corn-free shortening**
- **½ cup cane, beet or fruit sugar**
- **2½ cups sifted corn-free, self-rising flour**
- **1 teaspoon cinnamon**
- **½ teaspoon nutmeg**
- **¾ cup MILK**
- **½ cup raisins, rolled in flour**

Cream together shortening and sugar. Sift flour with spices. Alternately add milk and flour to creamed mixture. Mix well, then add floured raisins. Pour into a well-greased loaf tin. Bake in a preheated 350°F. oven for 35 to 45 minutes. Serves 8 to 10.

SPICE CAKE

- **1 cup cane, beet or fruit sugar**
- **6 tablespoons BUTTER**
- **1 cup BUTTERMILK**
- **1 teaspoon baking soda**
- **1 teaspoon vanilla**
- **2½ cups corn-free flour**
- **1 teaspoon nutmeg**
- **⅓ teaspoon ground cloves**
- **1 teaspoon cinnamon**
- **1 cup seedless raisins**

Cream sugar and butter. Add buttermilk (in which soda has been dissolved), vanilla, sifted dry ingredients and raisins. Grease and line with greased paper a square pan. Pour in batter. Bake in a 350°F. oven for about 45 minutes. Serves 8 to 10.

PINEAPPLE UPSIDE-DOWN CAKE

- **½ cup corn-free vegetable shortening**
- **½ cup cane, beet or fruit brown sugar, firmly packed**
- **1½ cups (No. 2 can) crushed pineapple, well drained**
- **¾ cup cane, beet or fruit sugar**
- **1½ cups sifted rye FLOUR**
- **¼ cup arrowroot**
- **1 tablespoon baking powder**
- **½ to ¾ teaspoon salt**
- **½ cup Mull-Soy**
- **½ cup water**

Melt ¼ cup at the shortening in a 9-inch square layer cake pan over low heat. Add brown sugar, stirring until it melts. Spread mixture evenly in bottom of pan and remove pan at once from heat. Arrange pineapple evenly on sugar mixture and set aside. Meanwhile, cream remaining ¼ cup shortening until fluffy. Gradually beat in sugar and continue beating until fluffy. Sift together rye flour, arrowroot, baking powder and salt. Combine Mull-Soy and water. Divide flour mixture into three parts. Divide Mull-Soy mixture into two parts. Add flour and the Mull-Soy portions alternately to the sugar mixture, starting and ending with the flour mixture, blending well after each addition. Turn batter into pan and spread evenly over pineapple. Bake in a 350°F. oven until the top center springs back when lightly touched with finger, about 45 to 50 minutes. Put cake pan upside down on serving plate and let stand a few minutes before removing pan. Serve cake hot or cold. Makes a 9-inch cake.

GINGERBREAD À LA GEORGIA

- ½ cup boiling water
- 1 cup molasses
- 2¼ cups rice or potato FLOUR
- 1 teaspoon baking soda
- ½ teaspoon salt
- 1½ teaspoons ginger
- 4 tablespoons olive oil

Add boiling water to molasses. Sift flour, soda, salt and ginger, then stir into molasses mixture. Add oil. Pour well-beaten batter into a greased shallow pan. Bake in a 350°F. oven for 30 minutes. Serves 8 to 10.

MRS. HOPE'S COFFEE CAKE

- ½ cup cane, beet or fruit sugar
- 3 tablespoons olive oil
- ½ cup soybean FLOUR
- ½ cup potato meal
- 1 tablespoon corn-free baking powder
- ½ teaspoon nutmeg (optional)
- ¾ teaspoon salt
- ⅔ cup coffee
- ¾ cup finely ground almonds
- 1 tablespoon fat
- 1 teaspoon cinnamon
- ½ cup brown cane, beet or fruit sugar

Mix sugar and oil well. Sift flour, potato meal, baking powder, nutmeg and salt. Add these alternately with the coffee. Pour into a well-greased pan. Cover with topping made from last four ingredients. Bake in a 400°F. oven for 20 to 25 minutes. Serve hot. Serves 6 to 8.

GINGERBREAD, NO. 1

- ½ cup boiling water
- ½ cup corn-free oil or vegetable shortening
- 1 cup dark molasses
- 2½ cups sifted corn-free flour
- 1 teaspoon baking soda
- ½ teaspoon salt
- 1½ teaspoons ginger
- 2 teaspoons corn-free baking powder

Pour boiling water over fat and molasses and blend until smooth. Sift dry ingredients together into molasses mixture, beating until free from lumps. Pour into large oblong pan, or layer pans that have been greased and lined with paper and greased again on the other side. Bake in a 375°F. oven for 25 to 30 minutes. Serves 8.

CLAUDIA'S CUPCAKES

- **1 cup cane, beet or fruit sugar**
- **2 cups rice FLOUR**
- **3 teaspoons corn-free baking powder**
- **½ teaspoon baking soda**
- **½ teaspoon salt**
- **½ teaspoon cloves**
- **1 teaspoon cinnamon**
- **½ cup cold coffee**
- **⅓ cup olive oil**
- **1 teaspoon vanilla**
- **½ cup chopped nuts**
- **1 cup finely chopped apple**

Sift first seven ingredients together. Stir in coffee, oil and vanilla. Blend in nuts and apple thoroughly. Put into greased muffin pans and bake in a 375°F. oven for 25 to 30 minutes. Makes 1 dozen.

RAISIN LOAF

- **1 cup dark brown cane, beet or fruit sugar**
- **⅓ cup corn-free oil**
- **1 cup raisins**
- **1 cup currants (or 2 cups raisins)**
- **½ teaspoon cloves**
- **1 teaspoon cinnamon**
- **½ teaspoon nutmeg**
- **¼ teaspoon allspice**
- **½ teaspoon salt**
- **1 cup water**
- **2 cups El Molino pastry whole-wheat FLOUR**
- **1 teaspoon corn-free baking powder**

Combine the first 10 ingredients mixing well. Cook 3 minutes then cool. Add flour, baking powder and mix well. Pour into a paper-lined loaf pan. Bake at 300°F. for 1 hour and 20 minutes. (If desired, ¾ cup chopped nuts may be added.) Makes 18 ½-inch pieces.

CHAMPION FRUITCAKE

- **1 cup raisins**
- **1 cup dates**
- **2 cups brown cane, beet or fruit sugar**
- **½ cup figs**
- **5 tablespoons soy BUTTER**
- **2 cups boiling water**
- **2 teaspoons cinnamon**
- **1 teaspoon cloves**
- **1 teaspoon baking soda**
- **1 teaspoon salt**
- **3 cups El Molino whole-wheat FLOUR (or pastry whole-wheat FLOUR)**
- **1 cup chopped pecans**
- **1 cup chopped walnuts**
- **1½ cups mixed candied fruit**
- **½ cup candied cherries**
- **½ cup diced citron**
- **Candied pineapple slices**

Combine the first five ingredients with boiling water. Let simmer over low fire for 10 minutes, then cool. Sift all dry ingredients with flour three times. Add pecans, walnuts, candied fruits and cherries, stirring well. Place in 9x5x2-inch loaf pan which has been well greased with corn-free oil and lined with greased paper. Decorate top with candied pineapple slices, nuts, cherries, citron, etc. Bake at 300°F. for 2 hours (or until done). Makes 4½ pound cake.

Note: For smaller cakes bake about 1 hour and 20 minutes. They will stay moist for a long time, if covered with a damp cloth.

SPICE CAKE WITH PINEAPPLE ICING (See recipe Part 11)

PINEAPPLE ICING (See recipe Part 11)

WHITE CAKE WITH SOY FLOUR (See recipe Part 11)

SPICY SUGAR CAKE (See recipe Part 11)

GINGERBREAD, NO. 2

1 cup shortening
4 cups sifted FLOUR
1 teaspoon cinnamon
1 teaspoon ginger
1 tablespoon baking soda
1 cup hot water
2 cups molasses

Melt shortening and pour over flour, mixing well. Add spices. Dissolve soda in hot water and add to flour with the molasses. Grease a biscuit pan and line with waxed paper, then grease again. Bake in a preheated 350°F. oven for 35 to 40 minutes. Serves 6 to 8.

GINGERBREAD, NO. 3

½ cup BUTTER
½ cup boiling water
1 teaspoon baking soda
1 cup molasses
2½ cups sifted FLOUR
¼ teaspoon salt
1½ teaspoons ginger

Melt butter. Combine with boiling water, in which soda has been dissolved, and molasses. When smooth, add sifted dry ingredients. Add to liquid, beating thoroughly. Grease an oblong tin and spread batter evenly. Bake in a 400°F. oven for 30 minutes. Serves 4 to 6.

Cookies

OATMEAL COOKIES

½ cup cane, beet or fruit sugar
¼ cup corn-free shortening
1 cup rolled oats
¼ cup MILK
¼ teaspoon baking soda
⅛ teaspoon nutmeg
⅛ teaspoon salt
1 cup corn-free cake flour
¼ teaspoon vanilla
½ cup raisins

Cream sugar and shortening. Add oats and milk, beating until creamy. Add soda, nutmeg, salt and flour. Add vanilla and raisins. Chill. Roll dough out thinly. Cut with cookie cutter. Bake in a 500°F. oven for 8 to 15 minutes. Makes 3 dozen small or 2 dozen large.

CAROB THINS

½ cup corn-free oil
3 tablespoons boiling water
1 tablespoon MILK
1 tablespoon honey
1 tablespoon lemon juice
1 cup El Molino whole-wheat FLOUR
1 cup El Molino unbleached white FLOUR
3 tablespoons carob powder
½ teaspoon salt

Place oil in a bowl and add boiling water and milk. Beat until it is thick and creamy. Add honey and lemon juice, beating well. Sift flours and salt and measure. Add carob powder and sift again. Turn into oil mixture, beating well. Form into loaf. Roll between two sheets of waxed paper, making sure the paper is no longer than the cookie sheet you will bake in. Carefully slip wax paper from top. Prick with fork and cut into 1½-inch squares. Slip paper and all onto cookie sheet. Bake in oven starting with 400°F., and after one or two minutes reduce to 350°F. for about 8 to 10 minutes. Makes 2 dozen.

Note: Watch carefully as these burn easily.

APRICOT BARS

1 cup sifted rice FLOUR
¼ cup CORNSTARCH
2 teaspoons baking powder
½ to ¾ teaspoon salt
1 cup brown sugar, firmly packed
¼ cup shortening, melted
1 cup diced dried apricots
¾ cup Mull-Soy

Sift together flour, cornstarch, baking powder and salt. Blend together sugar and shortening. Stir in apricots. Blend in dry ingredients. Gradually stir in Mull-Soy and mix until well blended. Turn batter into a greased 9x9x2-inch pan. Bake in a 375°F. oven for 25 to 30 minutes. Cool in pan. Remove from pan and cut into 1x2½-inch bars. Makes 24 bars.

OATMEAL DROP COOKIES

2 cups brown cane, beet or fruit sugar
1 cup margarine
4 cups rolled oats
1 level teaspoon salt
Rice FLOUR to mix soft dough
1 teaspoon cinnamon
1 teaspoon vanilla
1 teaspoon baking soda
½ cup boiling water

Mix ingredients, the soda dissolved in boiling water. Let stand until cold. Drop on greased tins. Bake in a preheated 450°F. oven for 10 to 12 minutes. Makes 10 dozen.

OATMEAL COOKIES, NO. 1 (See recipe Part 11)

OATMEAL COOKIES, NO. 2 (See recipe Part 11)

SOYALAC NUT CRESCENTS (See recipe Part 11)

DATE-COCONUT MACAROONS

3 tablespoons Soyalac (concentrated liquid)
4 dates, cut very fine
Pinch of salt
1 cup moist, sweetened coconut
½ teaspoon vanilla

Combine all ingredients. Drop by teaspoonfuls about 1 inch apart onto a cookie sheet covered with heavy brown wrapping paper. Bake in a 350°F. oven for about 8 minutes, or until lightly browned. Lift paper from baking sheet, place on damp towel for 2 minutes, then remove macaroons. Makes 1 dozen.

MOLASSES COOKIES

- **¼ cup olive oil**
- **¾ cup brown cane, beet or fruit sugar**
- **¼ cup molasses**
- **1 cup cooked and riced potatoes, salted**
- **1 cup potato flour**
- **¼ cup potato meal**
- **½ teaspoon baking soda**
- **¼ teaspoon salt**
- **1 tablespoon corn-free baking powder**
- **1 teaspoon vanilla**
- **2 teaspoons cinnamon**
- **¼ teaspoon nutmeg**
- **Raisins**

Mix oil, sugar, molasses and potatoes. Add potato flour, potato meal, soda, salt and baking powder. Add vanilla, cinnamon, nutmeg and a handful of raisins, mixing well. (Dough should be stiff.) Roll into small balls and place on greased cookie sheet. Press down with fork. Bake in a 375°F. oven for about 15 minutes. Makes 3 or 4 dozen.

COCONUT MACAROONS

- **1 (5.33-ounce) can condensed MILK**
- **1 (7-ounce) box shredded coconut**
- **¼ teaspoon vanilla**

Combine ingredients to form thick paste. Form into balls the size of a walnut. Drop on buttered tins. Bake in a preheated 350°F. oven for about 30 minutes. Makes about 15.

SUPERB EGGLESS COOKIES

- **½ pound sweet BUTTER**
- **5 tablespoons sugar**
- **1 tablespoon vanilla**
- **1 cup ground pecans**
- **2 cups FLOUR**
- **Pinch of salt**

Cream butter and sugar well. Add vanilla and nuts. Combine flour and salt and work in a little at a time. Form in small half-moon shapes. Bake in a preheated 350°F. oven for 15 to 20 minutes. Roll in sugar while still warm. Makes 2 dozen.

Pies

LEMON PIE

- **6 teaspoons Jolly Joan Egg Replacer**
- **6 tablespoons warm water**
- **1 cup cane, beet or fruit sugar**
- **¼ cup CORNSTARCH**
- **⅛ teaspoon salt**
- **1¼ cups hot water**
- **2 teaspoons grated lemon rind**
- **¼ cup lemon juice**
- **1 tablespoon corn-free oil**
- **1 9-inch baked pie crust**

Add egg replacer slowly to warm water in a mixing bowl. Mix thoroughly and whip with mixer until fluffy. In the top of a double boiler combine sugar, cornstarch and salt. Gradually pour in hot water, lemon rind and juice, stirring constantly over high heat. Place 3 tablespoons of mixture from double boiler into mixing bowl with egg replacer and beat until fluffy. Pour back into double boiler, and mix well. Add oil and continue stirring over high heat until smooth and thick enough to mound when dropped from a spoon. Cool 5 minutes. Pour into a baked pie shell and cool thoroughly. Serve plain or topped with whipped cream, if desired. Serves 8 to 10.

Puddings

SOYALAC WHIP

- **1 cup Soyalac**
- **2 teaspoons lemon juice**
- **⅛ teaspoon vanilla**
- **1 tablespoon cane, beet or fruit sugar**

Chill Soyalac. Whip in a deep bowl until quite thick. Add the remaining ingredients while continuing to whip. This may be used on fresh fruit or any desert where whipped cream is normally used. Serves 4.

SAUCES

REPLACER BATTER DIP

6 teaspoons Jolly Joan Egg Replacer

6 tablespoons warm water

Add Jolly Joan Egg Replacer slowly to warm water; mix thoroughly. Whip with mixer until fluffy. Dip pieces of chicken, steak, fish, oysters, shrimp, etc., in this mixture until thoroughly coated. It may be brushed on with a pastry brush if you prefer. Pan fry or deep fry in your favorite manner.

PART 10

No Egg, No Milk

BREADS

SOYALAC CORN BREAD (See recipe Part 12)

BREAD

1 tablespoon salt
1 tablespoon sugar
1 tablespoon chicken fat*
2 cups boiling water
½ envelope yeast
½ cup lukewarm water
6 to 6½ cups FLOUR

Put salt, sugar and chicken fat in mixing bowl large enough to allow for rising. Pour boiling water over mixture. Dissolve yeast in lukewarm water. When sugar mixture is cooled to lukewarm, add yeast, mix and stir well. Stir in flour. Knead dough until soft and elastic. Return to bowl, moisten, cover and let rise in warm place until doubled in bulk. Divide into loaves and place in greased pans. Cover and allow to double in bulk. Bake in a 450°F. oven for 1 hour. Makes 2 loaves.

*If not allergic to chicken

RYE BREAD
(Icebox)

¼ cup sugar
¼ cup vegetable oil
¼ cup boiling water
⅓ cup cold water
½ cake yeast
¼ cup lukewarm water
¼ teaspoon salt
1½ cups rye FLOUR
½ cup CORNSTARCH

Cream sugar and oil. Add boiling water and salt, mixing well. Add cold water. Dissolve yeast in lukewarm water and add to sugar-oil mixture. Sift flour and cornstarch together and add to sugar mixture. Refrigerate, covered, for at least 8 hours. Remove and shape dough into bread or rolls. Keep in a greased pan for at least 4 hours at 80°F. Preheat oven to 325° F. and bake bread 50 minutes; rolls 30 minutes. Makes 1 loaf or 2 dozen rolls.

RICE AND CORNMEAL MUFFINS

1½ cups rice FLOUR
⅔ cup CORNMEAL
2 tablespoons sugar
½ teaspoon salt
4 teaspoons baking powder
2 tablespoons shortening, melted
1 cup water

Sift all dry ingredients together. Add melted shortening and blend. Add water and beat for 3 to 5 minutes. Grease muffin tins. Bake in a preheated 350° F. oven for about 30 minutes. Makes 1 dozen.

SWEET POTATO MUFFINS

1 cup mashed sweet potatos
1 cup CORNMEAL
3 tablespoons sugar
1 teaspoon salt
2 tablespoons baking powder
1 cup dry rolled oats
3 tablespoons olive oil
¾ cup seedless raisins
¾ cup hot water

Mix well in order given. Bake in well-greased muffin pans in a 375°F. oven for about 20 minutes. (May be baked in loaf pan.) Makes 1 dozen.

MUFFINS

⅓ cup rice FLOUR
⅔ cup rye FLOUR
2 tablespoons baking powder
4 teaspoons cane, beet or fruit sugar
¼ teaspoon salt
⅔ cup water
½ teaspoon vegetable shortening, melted

After sifting dry ingredients together add water and shortening; beat thoroughly. Pour into muffin tins greased with vegetable shortening. Bake in a 400° F. oven for 25 minutes. Makes 6.

SALAD DRESSING

SOY MAYONNAISE (See recipe Part 5)

DESSERTS

Cakes

BART'S SPECIAL "COFFEE CAKE"

- **2 cups FLOUR**
- **1 teaspoon baking powder**
- **1 teaspoon salt**
- **1 cup brown sugar**
- **1¼ cups fruit juice (any kind)**
- **⅓ cup vegetable oil**
- **1 teaspoon nutmeg**
- **2 teaspoons cinnamon**
- **¼ teaspoon cloves**
- **¾ teaspoon raisins**
- **1 tablespoon water**

Grease and flour an 8x8x2-inch pan. Sift flour, baking powder and salt together. Combine sugar, fruit juice, oil, spices and raisins in a saucepan. Bring to a boil, boil 3 minutes and cool. Add sifted ingredients and water, then beat until smooth. Bake at 325°F. for 45 to 50 minutes. Makes 8 1-inch pieces or serves 6 to 8.

GINGERBREADS (See recipe Part 9)

CLAUDIA'S CUPCAKES (See recipe Part 9)

RAISIN LOAF (See recipe Part 9)

CHAMPION FRUITCAKE (See recipe Part 9)

PINEAPPLE UPSIDE-DOWN CAKE (See recipe Part 11)

SPICE CAKE WITH PINEAPPLE ICING (See recipe Part 11)

PINEAPPLE ICING (See recipe Part 11)

WHITE CAKE WITH SOY FLOUR (See recipe Part 11)

SPICY SUGAR CAKE (See recipe Part 11)

GINGERBREAD À LA GEORGIA (See recipe Part 9)

MRS. HOPE'S COFFEE CAKE (See recipe Part 9)

Cookies

DATE-COCONUT MACAROONS (See recipe Part 9)

MOLASSES COOKIES (See recipe Part 9)

OATMEAL COOKIES, NO. 1 (See recipe Part 11)

OATMEAL COOKIES, NO. 2 (See recipe Part 11)

SOYALAC NUT CRESCENTS (See recipe Part 11)

APRICOT BARS (See recipe Part 9)

OATMEAL DROP COOKIES (See recipe Part 9)

Puddings

SOYALAC WHIP (See recipe Part 9)

CAROB PUDDING (See recipe Part 13)

CORNSTARCH PUDDING (See recipe Part 13)

Candy

SOYALAC CAROB FUDGE (See recipe Part 13)

Ice Cream

ICE CREAM (See recipe Part 13)

VANILLA ICE CREAM (See recipe Part 13)

SAUCES

MUSHROOM SAUCE (MEAT) (See recipe Part 13)

PART 11

No Egg, No Wheat

BREADS

RYE BAKING POWDER BREAD

- 1½ cups whole rye FLOUR
- ½ teaspoon salt
- 5 teaspoons corn-free baking powder
- 4 teaspoons BUTTER, melted
- 1 cup MILK

Sift flour before measuring. Add salt and baking powder. Cut in butter. Beat in the milk. Bake in a 4x7-inch pan in a 375°F. oven for 25 minutes. Makes 1 loaf.

EGGLESS NUT BREAD

- 1½ cup Cellu wheatless mix
- 1 cup Cellu baking powder
- ⅛ teaspoon baking soda
- ¼ cup brown sugar
- 2 tablespoons molasses
- ¾ cup MILK
- ½ cup chopped walnuts

Combine dry ingredients in a bowl. Add molasses and milk, stirring until well blended. Add walnuts. Line bottom of an 8x4-inch loaf pan with wax paper and oil sides of pan. Pour dough into pan. Let stand in warm place for 20 minutes before baking. Bake in a preheated 350°F. oven for about 40 minutes.

Cover with aluminum foil for the first 20 minutes of baking time. Makes 1 small loaf.

BARLEY BREAD

1¾ cups whole barley flour
½ teaspoon salt
4½ teaspoons corn-free baking powder
1½ teaspoons soy margarine, melted
2 tablespoons honey
½ cup water

Sift flour before measuring. Combine dry ingredients and cut in margarine. Blend honey and water and add to dry ingredients. Bake in 4x7x2-inch pan at 375°F. for 25 minutes. Makes 1 loaf.

CORN BREAD

2 cups white CORNMEAL
1½ to 2 teaspoons salt
1 tablespoon baking powder
1 cup Mull-Soy
1 cup water
½ cup vegetable shortening, melted
3 tablespoons molasses

Combine cornmeal, salt and baking powder. Combine Mull-Soy, water, shortening and molasses. Pour all at once into cornmeal mixture and stir only until dry ingredients are dampened. Turn batter into greased 8x8x2-inch pan, spreading evenly with spoon or spatula. Bake in a 450°F. oven for about 20 minutes, or until it shrinks from sides of pan and is firm when touched lightly in center. Let cool in pan for 5 minutes. Remove and cut into 2-inch squares. Serve hot or cold. Makes 16 2-inch squares.

RYE AND CORNMEAL MUFFINS

⅓ teaspoon baking soda
1 cup BUTTERMILK
1 teaspoon baking powder
½ teaspoon salt
1 cup CORNMEAL
⅓ cup rye FLOUR
2 tablespoons BUTTER, melted

Dissolve soda in the buttermilk. Sift dry ingredients together. Add buttermilk and butter to the dry ingredients. Pour into greased muffin tins. Bake in a preheated 400°F. oven for 20 to 30 minutes. Makes 8 to 10.

CORNMEAL CAKES

1 cup boiling water
1 cup CORNMEAL
¼ teaspoon salt
1 teaspoon baking powder
1 teaspoon BUTTER, melted

Pour boiling water over mixed dry ingredients. Stir in butter. Drop by spoonfuls onto a greased skillet. Turn. Serve with corn syrup. Makes about 2 cups.

PANCAKES

1 cup sifted rice FLOUR
3 tablespoons sugar
2 tablespoons CORNSTARCH
½ to ¾ teaspoon salt
1½ teaspoons baking powder
⅓ cup Mull-Soy
⅔ cup water
3 tablespoons vegetable shortening, melted
CORN SYRUP

Sift together flour, sugar, cornstarch, salt and baking powder. Combine Mull-Soy, water and the slightly cooled melted shortening. Pour all at once into flour mixture, stirring until the mixture is smooth. For each pancake pour about 1 tablespoon of batter onto a preheated griddle. Bake until top surface is full of unbroken bubbles and under surface is golden brown. Turn with pancake turner and brown on other side. Serve at once with dark corn syrup. Makes 25.

Note: To test griddle for correct heat, pour a few drops of water on baking surface of griddle; if they dance in small beads, griddle is hot enough.

FISH

SALMON PATTIES

½ (15.5-ounce) can salmon
Salt and pepper to taste
4 tablespoons oatmeal
4 measures Nutramigen powder
Vegetable oil

Combine all the ingredients. Pat into desired shape. Brown well on each side in vegetable oil. Turn often until done. Serves 4.

SHRIMP GUMBO

1 tablespoon BUTTER
1 small onion, chopped (optional)
1 (12-ounce) can tomatoes
1 green pepper, seeded and minced
3 pieces chopped okra, minced
Minced parsley to taste
Minced celery to taste
½ teaspoon salt
⅛ teaspoon pepper (optional)
1 pound shrimp
½ cup vinegar
½ tablespoon CORNSTARCH

Melt butter. Brown onion (if allergic to onion, omit). Add tomatoes, minced vegetables, and salt and pepper. Boil shrimp in water to cover for 20 minutes. Drain shrimp and cover with vinegar. Shell shrimp, and remove veins. Add to tomato mixture. Thicken with cornstarch mixed in a little cold water. Serve over rice. Serves 4 to 6.

MEAT

MEAT LOAF (See recipe Part 9)

HAMBURGER PATTIE (See recipe Part 9)

POULTRY

POULTRY (See recipes Part 15)

POULTRY STUFFINGS

HOECAKE STUFFING (See recipe Part 9)

VEGETABLES

SCALLOPED CABBAGE

1 head cabbage
1 tablespoon BUTTER
1 cup MILK
1 tablespoon CORNSTARCH
CORNFLAKES

Cut cabbage into quarters. Cook until tender in boiling salted water, about 25 minutes. Make white sauce of butter, cornstarch and milk. Drain cabbage thoroughly and chop fine. Place in buttered baking dish. Pour white sauce over all and sprinkle with cornflakes. Bake at 400°F. for 20 minutes. Serve in baking dish. Serves 6.

PEAS AND MUSHROOMS

2 cups cooked peas
2 cups (or 1 pint) cooked fresh mushrooms
¼ cup CREAM
1 tablespoon CORNSTARCH
1 tablespoon BUTTER
½ teaspoon salt

Use canned or fresh peas. If fresh, shell and cook 20 to 30 minutes (depending on age of peas). Peel and wash mushrooms, cut up, cover with water and boil for 45 minutes. Add to peas. Drain remaining liquid from both vegetables. Thicken cornstarch with a little water, then blend in to the cream. Use less cornstarch if the liquid has cooked away. Melt butter while stirring in the vegetable. Add salt. Serve hot. Serves 6.

SALADS

RAW CARROT SALAD

3 carrots (about 1 cup)
1 teaspoon minced onion or parsley
¼ cup chopped peanuts
¼ cup chopped cucumber
Pickles, sweet or sour
Salt
Paprika
Eggless Salad Dressing*
Iceberg lettuce

Grate carrots using fine knife. Combine with onion, peanuts, cucumber, pickle and seasonings. Moisten generously with salad dressing. Chill and serve piled high on iceberg lettuce. Serves 2.

*See recipe under Salad Dressings, this part.

SALAD DRESSINGS

EGGLESS SALAD DRESSING

¾ teaspoon dry mustard
1 teaspoon salt
⅛ teaspoon pepper
¼ teaspoon celery salt
1 tablespoon CORNSTARCH
1 tablespoon sugar
1 cup CREAM
3 tablespoons vinegar or lemon juice

Combine dry ingredients and add cream in a saucepan. When smooth add boiling vinegar or lemon juice and cook until creamed.

Note: If inconvenient to use cream, ¾ cup MILK and ¼ tablespoon melted BUTTER may be substituted. Makes 20 tablespoons or 1½ cups.

RUSSIAN DRESSING

½ teaspoon salt
½ teaspoon dry mustard (optional)
¼ teaspoon paprika
¼ teaspoon sugar
Pinch of cayenne (optional)
3 tablespoons evaporated MILK
¾ cup salad oil
2 tablespoons vinegar or lemon juice

Mix together dry ingredients. Blend all with evaporated milk. Gradually beat in oil. Add vinegar or lemon juice. Beat until smooth. Makes 1 cup.

You may also add:

¼ cup chili sauce
1 tablespoon minced green pepper
1 tablespoon minced onion (or a pinch garlic salt)
1 tablespoon lemon juice

DESSERTS

Cakes

POTATO FLOUR EGGLESS CAKE

1 cup water
1 teaspoon baking soda
1 cup sugar
1 teaspoon cinnamon
1 teaspoon nutmeg
½ teaspoon cloves
½ teaspoon allspice
1 teaspoon baking powder
1½ cups potato flour
Pinch of salt
1 cup raisins
1 cup chopped nuts
1 cup BUTTER, melted

Bring water to boil and add soda. Mix the remaining ingredients, except the butter, thoroughly. Add butter. Place in well-greased cake tins and bake at 350°F. for 30 to 35 minutes, or until brown (or a straw that has been inserted is pulled out clean). Serves 10 to 12.

CAROB CAKE, NO. 1

½ cup corn-free shortening
1 cup carob powder
2 cups brown cane, beet or fruit sugar
2 cups potato flour
½ teaspoon salt
1 cup sour MILK
1 teaspoon vanilla
1½ teaspoons soda
½ cup boiling water
Creamy Carob Icing*

Cream shortening, carob and sugar. Sift together the flour and salt. Stir in milk and vanilla. Combine the soda and boiling water. Add the dry ingredients to the creamed mixture and then the soda and water. Grease two layer cake pans and pour in batter. Bake in a preheated 350°F. oven 30 minutes. Frost with Creamy Carob Icing. Serves 8 to 10.

*See recipe under Frostings, Part 15.

CAROB CAKE, NO. 2

½ cup corn-free shortening
2 cups brown cane, beet or fruit sugar
1 cup carob powder
2 cups wheat-free flour
½ teaspoon salt
1 cup sour MILK
1 teaspoon vanilla
1½ teaspoons soda
½ cup boiling water
Creamy Carob Icing*

Cream shortening, sugar and carob. Sift together flour and salt. Stir in milk and vanilla. Combine the soda and boiling water. Add the dry ingredients to the creamed mixture and then the soda and water. Grease two layer cake pans, and pour in batter. Bake in a preheated 350°F. oven for 30 minutes. Frost with Creamy Carob Icing. Serves 8 to 10.

*See recipe under Icings, Part 15.

SPICE CAKE WITH PINEAPPLE ICING

½ cup sugar
¼ cup vegetable shortening
½ cup Sobee liquid
½ cup water
½ teaspoon cinnamon
½ teaspoon mace
¼ teaspoon salt
½ teaspoon baking soda
½ teaspoon baking powder
¼ cup CORNSTARCH
1 cup sifted rye FLOUR
1 teaspoon vanilla
Pineapple Icing (recipe follows)

Cream together sugar and shortening. Add mixture of Sobee liquid and water. Combine cinnamon, mace, salt, soda, baking powder, cornstarch, flour and beat in. Add vanilla. Pour into an 8-inch layer pan. Bake in 375°F. oven for 25 to 30 minutes, or until cake is springy in the center. Serves 5 to 6.

PINEAPPLE ICING

- 4 tablespoons vegetable oil
- 2 cups confectioners' sugar
- 4½ cups crushed pineapple, well drained
- 5 to 6 tablespoons water
- 1 teaspoon vanilla
- 5 to 6 tablespoons Sobee liquid
- 2 to 3 drops yellow food coloring

Cream all ingredients well, adding food coloring. Cover spice cake top and sides.

WHITE CAKE WITH SOY FLOUR

- 3 tablespoons olive oil
- ¾ cup cane, beet or fruit sugar
- ⅔ cup soybean FLOUR
- ⅓ cup potato starch flour
- 1 tablespoon baking powder
- ½ teaspoon salt
- ½ teaspoon mace (or spice of your choice)
- ⅓ cup water
- 1 teaspoon almond flavoring or vanilla

Beat oil and sugar thoroughly. Sift dry ingredients. Add to oil-sugar mixture alternately with water. Add flavoring. Pour into a well-greased cake pan. Bake in a 375°F. oven for 30 to 35 minutes. Serves 6 to 8.

SPICY SUGAR CAKE

- 1½ cups potato flour
- ½ teaspoon baking soda
- ¾ cup potato meal
- 4½ teaspoons corn-free baking powder
- ½ teaspoon salt
- 1 tablespoon cinnamon
- ½ teaspoon spice of choice
- ½ cup olive oil
- 3 cups cane, beet or fruit sugar
- ¾ cup brown cane, beet, or fruit sugar
- 2¼ cups warm, sieved potatoes
- 1½ teaspoons vanilla or almond extract
- ½ cup carob powder

Sift the first seven ingredients and set aside. Cream oil and sugars. Add potato and flavoring. Beat well. Add the dry ingredients, a little at a time, mixing enough to blend well. Beat thoroughly. Line an oblong cake pan with aluminum foil. Smooth dough into pan and add carob. Bake in a 350°F. oven for 45 to 50 minutes. Serves 8 to 10.

YELLOW CAKE WHEAT-FREE

2 teaspoons Jolly Joan Egg Replacer
2 tablespoons warm water
1 cup cane, beet or fruit sugar
1 cup MILK
⅓ cup corn-free oil
1 teaspoon vanilla
1½ cups Jolly Joan Rice Mix

Add Jolly Joan Replacer slowly to warm water, mixing thoroughly. Beat until fluffy. Add sugar, mixing well. Add milk, oil and vanilla. Stir in Jolly Joan Rice Mix and beat until smooth. Pour into two 8-inch greased cake pans. Bake at 350°F. for 45 to 50 minutes. Frost, if desired. Serves 8.

ANNE'S GINGERBREAD

1 cup olive oil
2 cups brown sugar
1 cup water
3¾ cups potato flour
4 teaspoons ginger

Cream oil, sugar and gradually add water. Sift flour and ginger and add. Spread thin on a greased cookie sheet. Bake at 350°F. for 5 or 6 minutes, or until brown. Cut into squares before removing from pan. Makes about 3 dozen, depending on size.

Cookies

DATE-COCONUT MACAROONS (See recipe Part 9)

MOLASSES COOKIES (See recipe Part 9)

ALMOND COOKIES

1 cup rice FLOUR
½ cup light brown cane, beet or fruit sugar, packed
2 cups finely ground blanched almonds
6 tablespoons soy margarine, softened
1 tablespoon ice water
30 whole almonds

Sift flour and sugar together in a bowl. Blend in almonds. Work in margarine by hand. Stir in ice water. Break off tablespoon-sized pieces of dough and shape into balls. Put on greased cookie sheet 1 inch apart. Flatten slightly and place an almond in center of each. Bake in a 350°F. oven for 12 minutes. Makes 30.

OATMEAL COOKIES, NO. 1

2 cups oat flour
¾ cup fat
6 teaspoons confectioners' sugar
¾ teaspoon vanilla

Mix in order listed. Refrigerate for 1 hour. Drop on buttered cookie sheets. Bake at 400°F. for 30 minutes. Makes about 2 dozen.

OATMEAL COOKIES, NO. 2

2 cups brown sugar
1 cup shortening
4 cups rolled oats
1 level teaspoon salt
1 teaspoon baking soda
½ cup boiling water
1 teaspoon vanilla
CORNSTARCH

Blend sugar and shortening. Add oats, salt, soda dissolved in boiling water, vanilla and enough cornstarch to make a soft dough. Let mixture stand until thoroughly cold. Roll thin and cut into desired shapes. Bake on greased cookie sheets in a 500°F. oven for 8 to 12 minutes. Makes about 3 dozen.

SOYALAC NUT CRESCENTS

- **½ cup Soyalac (concentrated liquid)**
- **¼ cup CORNSTARCH**
- **2½ cups unsifted rice FLOUR**
- **1 cup vegetable shortening**
- **1 cup unsifted confectioners' sugar**
- **½ teaspoon salt**
- **1 tablespoon vanilla**
- **1½ cups chopped nuts (any allowed)**

Beat all ingredients, except nuts, until smooth and creamy, then add nuts. Chill dough. Shape into small crescents and place on an ungreased cookie sheet. Bake at 350°F. for 20 to 30 minutes, or until nicely browned. Crescents may be dusted with confectioners' sugar while still warm. Makes 5 dozen.

CHOCOLATE COCONUT MACAROONS

- **3 cups coconut**
- **1 (13-ounce) can condensed MILK**
- **2 ounces bitter chocolate, melted**
- **1 tablespoon CORN SYRUP**
- **1 teaspoon baking powder**

Combine coconut and milk and add chocolate. Sweeten with syrup. Add baking powder and mix well. Drop on buttered cookie sheet. Bake at 325°F. for 15 to 30 minutes. Place cookie sheet on a wet cloth before removing macaroons. Makes 2½ dozen, depending on size.

COCONUT MACAROONS

3 cups coconut
1 (13-ounce) can condensed MILK
1 teaspoon vanilla

Mix all ingredients. Make small cakes and place on a buttered cookie sheet. Bake at 350°F. for 15 to 20 minutes, or until brown. Place hot pan on a wet cloth to remove cookies easily. Makes 2½ to 3 dozen, depending on size.

CRISP COOKIES

½ cup vegetable shortening
½ cup cane, beet or fruit sugar
½ cup molasses
2 cups sifted rye FLOUR
2 teaspoons baking powder
¼ to ½ teaspoon salt
½ cup Mull-Soy
½ cup raisins or chopped prunes

Cream shortening and gradually beat in sugar. Continue beating until fluffy. Beat in molasses. Sift together flour, baking powder and salt. Divide flour mixture into three parts. Divide Mull-Soy into two parts. Add flour and Mull-Soy alternately to the sugar mixture, starting and ending with the flour. Blend well after each addition. Stir in raisins or prunes. Drop by teaspoonfuls, 3 inches apart, onto a greased cookie sheet. Bake in a 400°F. oven for about 8 minutes, or until edges are lightly browned. Remove from cookie sheet at once. Makes 4 dozen.

Puddings

RENNET CUSTARD (OR JUNKET)

1 cup MILK
⅛ cup sugar
½ tablespoon vanilla or
1 tablespoon wine (if allowed)
1 tablespoon liquid rennet

Heat milk, and when lukewarm, add sugar. Slowly add flavoring. When sugar is thoroughly dissolved, add rennet. Turn into mold and let cool until firm.

Note: Junket tablets may be substituted for rennet. Makes 1 cup or 2½ cups.

Dessert Sauces

JELLY SAUCE

4 ounces jelly
⅛ cup water
1 teaspoon BUTTER
1 teaspoon CORNSTARCH

Melt jelly in hot water, then add butter. Thin cornstarch with a little cold water and pour into jelly mixture. Cook until thick and smooth. Serve cold or hot over pudding. Makes ½ cup.

CHERRY SAUCE À LA RUSSE

1 (8-ounce) can bing cherries
CORNSTARCH
2 tablespoons sugar
Rum or brandy (if allowed)
French vanilla ICE CREAM

Drain cherries and measure juice. For each cup of juice add 1 tablespoon cornstarch and 2 tablespoons sugar, stirring to blend. Cook in the top of a double boiler, stirring until thickened. Add 2 tablespoons rum or brandy per cup of juice and cook for 10 minutes longer. While still hot, pour over hard, frozen homemade French vanilla ice cream. Makes 2 cups.

LEMON SAUCE

1 cup hot water
½ cup sugar
Juice and grated rind of ½ lemon
1 teaspoon CORNSTARCH
1 teaspoon BUTTER

Heat sugar, water, lemon juice and rind. Blend cornstarch with a little cold water and add to mixture. Add butter. When thick and smooth, remove from heat. Serve hot over pudding or cold on cake. Makes 1½ cups.

PART 12

No Egg, No Milk, No Wheat

BREADS

RICE AND RYE FLOUR BREAD

1⅓ cups rye FLOUR
⅔ cup rice FLOUR
½ teaspoon salt
2 tablespoons cane, beet or fruit sugar
3 generous tablespoons baking powder
2 teaspoons olive oil
1½ cups water

Sift dry ingredients together, then add oil and water, mixing well. Grease bread pans with oil and bake in a 350°F. oven for 40 minutes. Makes 1 loaf.

RYE BREAD

Sponge

1¼ cups warm water
1 cake yeast
2½ cups sifted rye FLOUR

Dough

2 teaspoons salt
2½ cups warm water
6½ cups sifted rye FLOUR

Mix sponge. Let stand (80°F.) until it breaks, about 2½ hours. For dough, dissolve salt in water. Add alternately with the flour to the sponge. Mix well and let rise in warm place (80°F.) about 30 minutes. When dough is light, divide into three loaves and place in greased pans. Moisten dough with a little water to prevent formation of a crust and let rise for about 1 hour. Bake in a 375°F. oven for about 1 hour. Makes 3 loaves.

SOYALAC CORN BREAD

1 cup Soyalac
1 cup water
¼ cup oil
3 tablespoons honey, molasses or sugar
2 cups yellow CORNMEAL
1½ teaspoons salt
1 tablespoon baking powder

Combine liquids, then blend dry ingredients. Pour liquids into the cornmeal mixture, stirring only until dry ingredients are dampened. Put batter into an oiled 8x8x2-inch pan, spreading evenly with spoon. Bake at 450°F. for about 20 minutes, or until center top is firm when touched lightly. Allow to cool for 5 minutes before cutting into 2-inch squares and removing from pan. Serve hot or cold. Serves 4.

SOUTHERN CORN PONE

⅓ teaspoon salt
¼ cup CORNMEAL
½ cup boiling water

Sift dry ingredients and scald with boiling water. Drop on well-greased pan (using peanut oil or bacon grease). Bake in a preheated 400°F. oven for 8 minutes, or until brown. Makes 4 small cakes.

CROUTONS

Pack commercial hominy mush in an ice-cube tray. Chill, but do not freeze. Cut into ¼-inch slices and slice in ¼-inch squares.

Dip in CORNMEAL, then fry in deep chicken fat or other butter substitute.

CINNAMON TOAST

4 rye (or wheat-free) crackers
Margarine
2 tablespoons cane, beet or fruit sugar
1 tablespoon cinnamon

Heat crackers and spread with margarine. Combine sugar and cinnamon and sprinkle on top of crackers. Serves 2 to 4.

RICE MUFFINS

¼ cup vegetable shortening
¼ cup cane, beet or fruit sugar
1 teaspoon salt
¼ cup CORNSTARCH
2 tablespoons baking powder
1 cup Sobee liquid
1 cup rice FLOUR
1 cup water
1 cup rice cereal

Beat shortening, sugar, salt, cornstarch and baking powder until smooth and creamy. Add Sobee liquid and rice flour alternately, beating until smooth after each addition. Stir in water. Add rice cereal and stir lightly. Fill greased muffin tins two-thirds full. Bake in a 400°F. oven for 25 to 30 minutes, or until brown. Makes 1 dozen.

SOYALAC PANCAKES

½ cup Soyalac
½ cup water
2 tablespoons vegetable oil
1 cup sifted rice FLOUR
2 tablespoons cane, beet or fruit sugar or molasses
2 tablespoons CORNSTARCH
½ teaspoon salt
1½ teaspoons baking powder

Combine liquid ingredients and blend in dry ingredients, stirring until mixture is smooth. Bake in small cakes on preheated griddle until each cake is full of bubbles and the undersurface is brown. Turn and brown on other side. Serve while hot with syrup. Makes 6 to 8.

SOYALAC CORN STICKS

1 cup yellow CORNMEAL
½ cup Soyalac
½ cup water
½ teaspoon salt
1 tablespoon brown sugar
1 tablespoon oil

Combine all the ingredients and refrigerate for 30 minutes. Pour into iron corn-stick pans that have been oiled and are very hot. Bake at 400°F. for 20 minutes. Makes 8.

CEREALS

CORNMEAL MUSH

½ cup CORNMEAL
½ teaspoon salt
2 cups water

Stir the cornmeal and salt into the rapidly boiling water. Transfer to the top of a double boiler and cook for 1 hour. Makes 3 cups.

GRITS

4 cups water
1 cup grits
½ teaspoon salt

Stir the grits and salt into the boiling water. Transfer to the top of a double boiler and cook for 1 hour. Makes 5 cups.

Note: An instant hominy grits is on the market.

OATMEAL (See recipe Part 15)

"Instant" cereals might have allergenics, so use only if permissible.

SOUPS

CHICKEN SOUP

1 (3- to 4-pound) fowl
1 tablespoon salt
3 to 4 quarts cold water
1 onion (optional)
2 stalks celery
¼ cup diced celery
¼ teaspoon pepper (optional)
CORNSTARCH sauce (optional)

Singe, clean and cut up fowl. Salt and let stand for several hours. Cover with cold water and bring to a boil quickly. Skim thoroughly. Simmer 3 hours or longer. Add the vegetables and boil 1 hour more. Strain, and season soup to taste. Cut up chicken for salads, croquettes, or serve with cornstarch sauce. Serves 4 to 6.

MEATS

LENTIL MEAT LOAF

1 pound ground round beef
2 cups cooked lentils, mashed
1 cup cooked rice
½ cup chopped celery
⅔ cup Soyalac
1 teaspoon salt
½ teaspoon sage
⅔ cup water

Combine all ingredients and mix well. Bake in oiled casserole at 350°F. for 45 minutes. Serve with tomato gravy. Makes 6½ cups.

MEAT-RICE PATTIES

½ pound ground beef
¾ cup cooked rice
½ to ¾ teaspoon salt
¼ cup Mull-Soy

Combine all ingredients. Shape into patties, using ¼ cup mixture for each patty. Place on broiler pan, 3 inches from heat and cook until browned. Turn and brown the other side. Serve hot. Makes 6.

POULTRY STUFFINGS

HOECAKE STUFFING (See recipe Part 9)

SWEDISH STUFFING

2 bouillon cubes*
3 cups hot water
1¼ teaspoons sage
3 stalks celery, chopped
1½ onions, chopped (optional)
¼ teaspoon pepper
2 teaspoons salt
2 teaspoons dried parsley
8 cups Swedish rye crumbs

Dissolve bouillon cubes in hot water. Stir in sage, pepper, salt and parsley, celery and onion. Combine with crumbs and mix thoroughly. Makes 12 cups.

*Read label carefully for wheat content.

RICE DRESSING

2 tablespoons diced onion
2 tablespoons fat (chicken fat preferably)
1 cup chopped celery
2 teaspoons Worcestershire sauce
2 cups cooked rice
½ teaspoon salt
1/16 teaspoon pepper (or paprika)

Brown onion in fat. Add to remaining ingredients and blend thoroughly. Stuff fowl or breast of veal. Pin together with skewers. Makes 3 cups.

DESSERTS

Cakes

SPICE CAKE WITH PINEAPPLE ICING (See recipe Part 11)

PINEAPPLE ICING (See recipe Part 11)

WHITE CAKE WITH SOY FLOUR (See recipe Part 11)

SPICY SUGAR CAKE (See recipe Part 11)

PINEAPPLE UPSIDE-DOWN CAKE

½ cup corn-free vegetable shortening
½ cup brown cane or beet sugar, firmly packed
1½ cups (No. 2 can) crushed pineapple, well drained
¾ cup granulated cane, beet or fruit sugar
1½ cups sifted rye FLOUR
¼ cup arrowroot
1 tablespoon baking powder
½ to ¾ teaspoon salt
½ cup Mull-Soy
½ cup water

Melt ¼ cup of the shortening in 9-inch square layer cake pan over low heat. Add brown sugar and stir until it melts. Spread mixture evenly over bottom of pan and remove at once from heat. Arrange pineapple evenly over sugar mixture and set aside. Meanwhile, cream the remaining ¼ cup shortening until fluffy.

Gradually beat in granulated sugar until fluffy. Sift together flour, arrowroot, baking powder and salt. Combine Mull-Soy and water. Divide flour mixture into two parts. Add flour and the Mull-Soy portions alternately to the sugar mixture, starting and ending with the flour mixture, blending well after each addition. Turn batter into prepared pan, spreading evenly over pineapple. Bake in a 350°F. oven for about 45 to 50 minutes, or until top center springs back when lightly touched with finger. Put cake pan upside down on serving plate and let stand a few minutes before removing pan. Serve cake hot or cold. Makes one 9-inch cake.

GINGERBREAD, NO. 1

- **4 tablespoons soy shortening**
- **2 tablespoons molasses**
- **½ teaspoon ginger**
- **¼ teaspoon cinnamon**
- **¼ teaspoon salt**
- **½ cup plus 1 tablespoon boiling water**
- **1 cup Cellu rye flour**
- **⅛ teaspoon corn-free baking soda**
- **4 teaspoons corn-free baking powder**

Combine shortening, molasses, spices and salt in a bowl and add boiling water. Sift flour, baking powder and soda into mixture and beat. Pour into 9x5x2-inch or 8x8-inch greased loaf pan and bake at 350°F. for 40 minutes. Serves 8.

WHITE CAKE WITH SOY FLOUR

- **3 tablespoons suet, melted**
- **¾ cup cane, beet or fruit sugar**
- **⅔ cup soybean FLOUR**
- **⅓ cup potato starch flour**
- **3 teaspoons corn-free baking powder**
- **½ tablespoon salt**
- **½ teaspoon mace**
- **⅓ cup water**
- **1 teaspoon vanilla**

Combine suet and sugar. Add dry ingredients alternately with the water. Add vanilla and beat well. Put into a 9-inch pan greased with corn-free fat. Bake at 375°F. for 30 to 35 minutes, or until straw inserted comes out clean. Serves 6 to 8.

WHITE CAKE WITH RICE FLOUR

- **¾ cup cane, beet or fruit sugar**
- **3 tablespoons suet, melted**
- **⅔ cup rice FLOUR**
- **⅓ cup potato starch flour**
- **3 teaspoons corn-free baking powder**
- **½ teaspoon salt**
- **½ teaspoon mace**
- **⅓ cup water**
- **1 teaspoon vanilla**

Blend sugar and suet well. Sift dry ingredients. Combine the first two mixtures with the water, beating well. Add vanilla last. Put into a 9-inch pan greased with corn-free fat. Bake in a 375°F. oven for 30 to 35 minutes, or until straw inserted comes out clean. Serves 6 to 8.

GINGERBREAD, NO. 2

- **1 cup corn-free molasses**
- **½ cup boiling water**
- **2¼ cups rice FLOUR (or ½ rice and ½ potato flour)**
- **1 teaspoon corn-free baking powder**
- **1½ teaspoons ginger**
- **½ teaspoon salt**
- **4 tablespoons corn-free margarine, melted**

Blend molasses and water. Sift dry ingredients and add to molasses. Stir in margarine, beating well. Pour into a 9-inch shallow pan greased with corn-free margarine. Bake in a 350°F. oven for about 30 minutes. Serves 6 to 8.

BROWN SUGAR SPICE CAKE

- **½ cup corn-free vegetable shortening**
- **½ cup cane, beet or fruit sugar**
- **½ cup brown cane, beet or fruit sugar**
- **½ teaspoon salt**
- **1 teaspoon cinnamon**
- **½ teaspoon mace**
- **1 teaspoon baking soda**
- **1 teaspoon corn-free baking powder**
- **¾ cup Sobee liquid**
- **2 cups sifted rice FLOUR**
- **½ cup water**
- **½ cup white raisins**
- **½ cup chopped nuts (if permitted in diet)**
- **1 teaspoon vanilla**

Cream first six ingredients together. Add baking soda and baking powder. Add alternately, beginning and ending with flour, the Sobee liquid and 1 cup flour. Beat until smooth. Gradually add the water and the remaining 1 cup flour (save a small portion of flour to mix with raisins). Stir in raisins, nuts and vanilla. Pour into a well-greased 9-inch cake pan. Bake at 375°F. for 30 minutes. Test with toothpick. Serves 8 to 10.

BIRTHDAY CAKE

- **1¼ cups potato flour**
- **½ cup potato meal**
- **¼ teaspoon salt**
- **2 tablespoons corn-free baking powder**
- **¼ teaspoon baking soda**
- **½ cup corn-free fat, melted**
- **1½ cups cane, beet or fruit sugar**
- **1½ cups salted, hot riced potatoes**
- **½ cup plain or caramelized cane, beet or fruit sugar**

Sift the first five ingredients. Cream the last four ingredients. Add the flour mixture, mixing just enough to blend well. Pour the batter into an 8x8-inch pan, well greased with corn-free fat. Bake at 350°F. for about 35 to 40 minutes. Cool before turning out of pan. Makes 12 cupcakes.

SPICY SUGAR CAKE (See recipe Part 11)

Cookies

OATMEAL COOKIES, NO. 1 (See recipe Part 11)

OATMEAL COOKIES, NO. 2 (See recipe Part 11)

SOYALAC NUT CRESCENTS (See recipe Part 11)

Pie

RYE AND CORNSTARCH CRUST

¾ cup rye FLOUR
¼ cup CORNSTARCH or rice flour
⅓ cup chicken fat or margarine
2 tablespoons cold water (approximate)

Sift together flour, cornstarch. Mix with shortening. Add enough cold water to hold together. Put cornstarch on board and roll. Makes 1 9-inch crust.

Puddings

APRICOT FLUFF

Make as Banana Fluff*, substituting apricots for bananas.

*See recipe under Puddings, Part 3.

PRUNE PUDDING

1 cup prunes
1 cup cold water
½ cup CORN SYRUP
Juice and grated rind of ½ lemon
1-inch stick cinnamon
1¾ cups boiling water
⅓ cups CORNSTARCH

Soak prunes in cold water for 1 hour, then boil until soft. Drain and remove stones. Add syrup, lemon juice and rind, cinnamon and boiling water. Simmer for 15 minutes. Mix cornstarch with enough cold water to pour easily. Add to prunes and cook 5 minutes longer. Remove cinnamon stick. Place in mold and chill. Serves 4.

INDIAN PUDDING

¼ cup yellow CORNMEAL
¼ cup water
1 cup Mull-Soy
1 cup boiling water
½ cup raisins or finely cut prunes
½ cup molasses

Combine cornmeal and ¼ cup water in the top of a double boiler. Let stand for 5 minutes. Stir in Mull-Soy and then the boiling water. Cook over boiling water, stirring often, until thickened, about 20 minutes. Stir in raisins or chopped prunes and molasses. Pour into greased 1-quart casserole or baking dish. Bake in a 325°F. oven for 2 hours. Serve hot. Serves 4 to 6.

APPLE TAPIOCA

¾ cup pearl tapioca
2½ cups boiling water
½ teaspoon salt
7 sour apples
½ cup sugar
CORNSTARCH Fruit sauce*

Soak tapioca in cold water to cover for 1 hour. Drain. Add boiling water and salt. Cook in the top of a double boiler until transparent. Core and peel apples. Arrange apples in greased pudding dish and fill cavities with sugar. Pour tapioca over. Bake in a 400°F. oven for 30 minutes, or until apples are soft. Serve with Fruit sauce. Serves 8.

*See recipe, this part under Sauces.

SAUCES

FRUIT SAUCE

2 tablespoons brown sugar
1 cup fruit juice (pineapple, cherry, peach, apricot, etc.)
1 teaspoon CORNSTARCH

Heat sugar and juice. Mix cornstarch with a little juice and add to juice, stirring until smooth. Cook about 10 minutes. Serve warm on steamed pudding. Makes about 1 cup.

CORNSTARCH FRUIT SAUCE

1 cup sugar
Juice and grated rind of 1 lemon
2 tablespoons CORNSTARCH
2 cups boiling water

Combine sugar, lemon juice and rind and cornstarch with boiling water. Cook 8 to 10 minutes, adding water to maintain quantity. Serve hot. Makes about 3 cups.

HORSERADISH SAUCE

¼ onion, finely chopped
1 tablespoon peanut oil
3 tablespoons grated horseradish
1 cup chicken or beef soup stock
1 tablespoon brown sugar
2 cloves
2 bay leaves
Salt and pepper
2 tablespoons vinegar
1 tablespoon CORNSTARCH

Brown onion in the oil in a frying pan. Add 2 tablespoons of the horseradish, soup stock, sugar, cloves, bay leaves, salt and pepper and vinegar. Thicken with cornstarch which has been blended with a little cold soup stock. Add rest of horseradish. Cook a few minutes, then add more sugar or vinegar, if necessary. Remove bay leaves before serving. Serve with beef chuck. Makes about 1½ cups.

SAUCE FOR ASPARAGUS

1 cup asparagus liquid
Salt and pepper (optional)
1 tablespoon CORNSTARCH

Cook fresh asparagus until tender or use canned asparagus. Reserve 1 cup liquid. Heat and season to taste with salt and pepper. Add cornstarch to a little liquid and thicken. Pour over hot asparagus. Makes about 1 cup.

SAUCE FOR CAULIFLOWER

1 cup cauliflower liquid
1 tablespoon CORNSTARCH
CORNFLAKES

Save 1 cup liquid in which cauliflower has been cooked. Blend cornstarch with a little of the liquid. Heat remaining liquid, adding cornstarch mixture a little at a time. Pour over cauliflower and sprinkle cornflakes on top. Brown in oven. Makes about 1 cup.

SAUCE FOR CHICKEN

Chicken "leavings" (pieces left in pan)
1 cup hot water
Crushed CORNFLAKES
1 tablespoon CORNSTARCH
2 teaspoons chopped parsley
Salt and pepper (optional)

After chicken has been fried, remove to platter. Add 1 cup hot water to skillet and a scooping of cornflakes. Boil. Add cornstarch to a little cold water. Pour into boiling mixture and thicken. Add parsley, salt and pepper. Pour over fried chicken. Serve hot. Makes about 1 cup.

SAUCE SOY

1½ cups water
1½ tablespoons CORNSTARCH
1 tablespoon soy sauce
3 bouillon cubes

Blend water and cornstarch. Add soy sauce and bouillon cubes. Cook over low heat, stirring constantly, until mixture is thickened and translucent. Serve over hot Rice Pancakes (see recipe Part 8) or any other dish of your choice. Makes about 1½ cups.

SECTION III

MILK ALLERGY

INTRODUCTION

Milk may likely be the first allergen in a person's life because he starts on some kind of milk on Life Day One. Later on milk is "hidden" in so many foods, as are corn, wheat and eggs, that one can develop an allergy to milk later in life. Sometimes milk allergy may seem to suddenly appear soon after one develops his ulcer and starts living with milk or cream diet, much as one may develop hay fever in an unusual pollen season.

Milk has two protein fractions; casein and lactalbumin and the latter is much more responsible for allergy. Cow's and goat's milk contain the same casein fraction but a different lactalbumin, which is why goat's milk can often be used successfully to replace cow's milk in an allergic person.

Cheese is a form of milk, but it is also different because of its other components. One can still be allergic to a specific cheese although milk is totally innocent as an offender. Casein is the curd fraction of milk. Cheeses made from the curd can often be eaten by a milk allergic person. Common cheeses containing or made from lactalbumin (whey) such as cottage or cream cheese will cause more trouble in the milk allergic.

Look out for powdered milk and casein, margarine may contain milk solids. When in doubt take the label to your doctor.

The following list shows most of the possible contacts with milk:

Milk Allergy—Introduction

Baker's bread**
Baking powder biscuits
Bavarian cream
Bisques

Blanc mange
Boiled salad dressings
Bologna
Butter
Buttermilk
Butter sauces
Cakes
Candies, except hard or home-made
Cheeses of every description*
Chocolate or cocoa drinks or mixtures
Chowders
Cooked sausages
Cookies
Cream
Creamed foods
Cream sauces
Curd
Custards
Doughnuts
Eggs
Flour mixtures
Foods, prepared au gratin
Foods fried in butter; fish, poultry, beef or pork
Fritters
Gravies
Hamburgers**
Hard sauces
Hash
Hotcakes
Ice creams
Junket
Malted milk
Mashed potatoes
Meat loaf
Milk chocolate
Milk, which includes—condensed, dried, evaporated, fresh, goat's, malted milk and powdered milk
Oleomargarines
Omelets
Ovaltine
Ovomalt
Pie crust made with milk products
Popcorn
Popovers
Prepared flour mixtures, such as: biscuit, cake, cookies, doughnuts, muffins, pancake, pie crust, waffles and puddings
Rarebits
Salad dressings, "boiled"
Scrambled and escalloped dishes
Sherbets
Soda crackers
Soufflés
Soups
Milk or cream
Spanish cream
Spumoni
Waffles
Whey
Yogurt
Zwieback

*Although all cheeses are to be considered as milk products, a patient not sensitive to milk may be found allergic to one or more cheeses. Therefore, consider each kind and brand of cheese as a separately specific allergen.

**Not all preparations of these contain milk. Check and read! Kosher breads are milk free.

When you inquire concerning the presence of milk in any product, put your question in this way: "Do you use butter, oleomargarine, cream, cheese of any kind, fresh milk, buttermilk, dried milk, powdered milk, condensed milk, evaporated milk, or yogurt in this food?"

Note: Be sure all margarines and butter in milk recipes are soy margarine or butter, if not allergic to soy products.

PART 13

NO MILK

BREADS

DATE AND WALNUT BREAD

- 2 teaspoons baking soda
- 1½ cups boiling water
- 2 EGGS, separated
- ½ cup cane, beet or fruit sugar
- 2 tablespoons corn-free shortening, melted
- 2 teaspoons vanilla
- 1 pound dates, cut into quarters
- Pinch of salt
- 3½ cups sifted corn-free flour
- 1 scant teaspoon corn-free baking powder
- ½ cup chopped walnuts
- Raisins

Dissolve soda in boiling water. Separate eggs and beat yolks with sugar. Add soda. Stir in shortening and vanilla. Add dates to mixture. Beat egg whites until stiff, adding a pinch of salt. Fold into mixture. Add the remaining ingredients in order. Bake in two well-greased loaf pans in a 300°F. oven for 1 to 1½ hours. Makes 2 loaves.

ORANGE BREAD

- **2 tablespoons shortening**
- **¼ cup cane, beet or fruit sugar**
- **1 EGG**
- **1½ cups all-purpose, corn-free flour**
- **3 teaspoons corn-free baking powder**
- **½ teaspoon salt**
- **½ cup minced candied orange rind**
- **½ cup coconut milk**
- **¼ cup orange juice**

Cream shortening, adding sugar gradually. Add egg and beat until light. Sift dry ingredients together. Blend in orange rind. Add to shortening mixture alternately with coconut milk. Add orange juice last. Pour into well-greased 9x5x2-inch loaf pan. Allow to stand 20 minutes. Bake in a 350°F. oven for about 45 minutes to 1 hour. Makes 1 medium-sized loaf.

QUICK-RAISED RICE BREAD

- **2 EGGS, separated, or 2 teaspoons Jolly Joan Egg Replacer plus 2 tablespoons water**
- **1 cup soy milk**
- **2 tablespoons corn-free oil**
- **2 tablespoons corn-free sugar**
- **2 cups Jolly Joan Rice Mix**

Beat whites until stiff. In a separate bowl beat egg yolks, then add milk, oil and sugar. Add rice mix and stir until smooth. Gently fold in egg whites until batter is mixed. Pour into a 8x4x2-inch bread pan. Bake in a preheated 350°F. oven for 45 minutes, or until brown. Turn out on wire rack until cool. Makes 1 loaf.

BAKING POWDER BISCUITS

2 cups corn-free flour
4 teaspoons baking powder
½ teaspoon salt
2 tablespoons shortening (chicken fat or vegetable margarine)
⅔ to ¾ cup MILK or coconut milk

Sift together dry ingredients. Add shortening, mixing with fork. Add milk. Roll or pat on floured board to a ½-inch thickness. Cut with biscuit cutter that has been dusted with flour. Bake in a preheated 475°F. oven for 10 to 12 minutes. Makes about 15.

Note: This recipe can be varied by adding 1 tablespoon sugar and ½ cup chopped, seeded raisins to dough.

COCONUT PANCAKES

1¼ cups rice FLOUR
¼ teaspoon salt
1½ cups beet, cane or fruit sugar
4 EGGS
3 cups coconut milk
½ cup corn-free cooking oil

Sift flour, salt and sugar into a bowl. Beat in eggs and coconut milk until very smooth. Heat 2 teaspoons of oil in a skillet. Lightly brown each pancake on both sides. Roll up like a jelly roll. Keep warm in a bun warmer. Repeat for each pancake. Makes about 2½ dozen.

RICE SHEET BREAD

- **1 cup Cellu soybean flour**
- **¾ cup Cellu rice flour**
- **4 teaspoons Cellu baking powder**
- **¼ teaspoon salt**
- **3 tablespoons cane, beet or fruit sugar**
- **¼ cup corn-free fat, melted**
- **1 cup plus 2 tablespoons cold water**

Combine ingredients in order given. This makes a medium-thin batter. Pour batter (which should not exceed a ¼-inch thickness) into an 8x8-inch baking pan greased with corn-free fat. Bake at 400°F. for about 1 hour. Serves 6 to 8.

RYE MUFFINS

- **1 cup sifted rye FLOUR**
- **2 teaspoons corn-free baking powder**
- **¼ to ½ teaspoon salt**
- **¼ cup Mull-Soy**
- **¼ cup water**
- **2 tablespoons corn-free margarine, melted**
- **2 tablespoons molasses**

Sift together the flour, baking powder and salt. Combine Mull-Soy, water, fat and molasses. Pour Mull-Soy mixture, all at once, into dry ingredients and stir until dry ingredients are moistened. Turn batter into well-greased 2-inch muffin cups, filling two-thirds full. Bake in a 400°F. oven for 25 to 30 minutes, or until tops are browned. Makes 6 medium-sized muffins.

SOYALAC CORN BREAD (See recipe Part 12)

BARLEY BREAD (See recipe Part 11)

CORNBREAD (See recipe Part 11)

RYE AND CORNMEAL MUFFINS (See recipe Part 11)

CORNMEAL CAKES (See recipe Part 11)

PANCAKES (See recipe Part 11)

RICE AND RYE FLOUR BREAD (See recipe Part 12)

RYE BREAD (See recipe Part 12)

SOUTHERN CORN PONE (See recipe Part 12)

CROUTONS (See recipe Part 12)

CINNAMON TOAST (See recipe Part 12)

RICE MUFFINS (See recipe Part 12)

SOYALAC CORN STICKS (See recipe Part 12)

SOYALAC PANCAKES (See recipe Part 12)

SOUTHERN ROLLS

½ cup soy margarine
½ cup cane, beet or fruit sugar
2 teaspoons salt
1 cup hot mashed potatoes (about 3 medium-sized potatoes)
1 EGG, beaten
2 cups water
1 cake compressed yeast
6 cups sifted FLOUR

Blend margarine, sugar and salt into the potatoes. Stir in the egg. Boil water and cool to lukewarm. Add the water to the potatoes, alternating with 2 cups flour. Beat hard. Dissolve yeast in ¼ cup of batter. Mix all well. Cover with kitchen towel and let rise 30 minutes in a warm place. Add 6 cups flour (measured after sifting) to batter. Knead well for 5 minutes. Return dough to bowl and cover. Let rise until doubled in bulk, about 1½ to 2 hours. Roll dough out to a ½-inch thickness. Cut into rounds with a large biscuit cutter. With a dull knife press through center of round and fold in half. Pinch edges of roll together and place in greased pan. Let rise again for 2 hours. Bake in a 450°F. oven for 20 to 30 minutes. Makes about 30.

NUT AND PRUNE BREAD

¾ cup chopped nuts
¾ cup cooked prunes, cut up
1 cup sifted white FLOUR
1 teaspoon salt
2 tablespoons baking powder
½ cup cane, beet or fruit sugar
3 cups graham FLOUR
1 teaspoon cinnamon
1½ cups prune juice
½ cup fat, melted
1 EGG

Add nuts and prunes to dry ingredients. Stir in prune juice, then fat and egg, mixing well. Pour mixture into a greased bread pan. Bake in a 350°F. oven for 1 hour and 15 minutes. Makes 1 loaf.

POTATO FLOUR OR TAPIOCA FLOUR MUFFINS

4 EGGS, separated
¼ teaspoon salt
1 tablespoon cane, beet or fruit sugar
2 tablespoons ice water
½ cup Cellu potato flour or Cellu tapioca flour
1 teaspoon Cellu baking powder

Beat egg yolks with salt and sugar. Add water. Sift flour and baking powder together and add to egg mixture. Stiffly beat egg whites and fold in. Pour into greased muffin pans. Bake in a 360°F. oven for 15 to 20 minutes. Makes 6 to 8 large muffins.

CEREAL

CORNMEAL MUSH (See recipe Part 12)

GRITS (See recipe Part 12)

OATMEAL (See recipe Part 12)

CEREALS COOKED IN MULL-SOY

1½ cups water
½ cup Mull-Soy
¼ to ½ teaspoon salt
½ cup allowed cereal (such as CORNMEAL, farina, rice)

Combine water, Mull-Soy and salt in the top of a double boiler. Heat to a brisk boil. Slowly stir in cereal. Boil gently for 3 to 5 minutes, stirring constantly. Cover and cook over boiling water, stirring once in a while, for 30 minutes. Makes 3 servings.

Note: If cereal is for a young infant, increase cooking time over boiling water to 45 to 50 minutes. Strain before serving.

INDIVIDUAL SHORTCAKES

2 cups FLOUR
1 tablespoon baking powder
½ teaspoon salt
4 tablespoons shortening
1 EGG
½ cup water

Sift together dry ingredients. Cut in shortening. Add egg and enough water to make soft dough. Half fill greased muffin rings. Bake in a preheated 475°F. oven for 10 to 12 minutes. Split and fill with hot creamed mushrooms or chicken. Serves 4 to 6.

Note: To use with fruit as shortcake, add 1 tablespoon sugar to dry ingredients before sifting.

SOUPS

CREAMED TOMATO SOUP

1 cup thin Basic Cream Sauce made with Soyalac*
1 cup tomato juice
Salt to taste

Heat the cream sauce and tomato juice separately, then stir the tomato juice slowly into the cream sauce—do not boil. Serve at once. Makes 2 cups.

*See recipe under Sauces, this part.

BASIC CREAM SOUP

1½ or 2 cups any canned or frozen vegetable
1 cup thin Basic Cream Sauce* (using the thickening agent that is allowed)
Salt and pepper

Liquefy vegetables or put through a coarse sieve. Add to the cream sauce. Season to taste and serve hot. Makes 2½ to 3 cups.

*See recipe under Sauces, this part.

TOMATO CREAM SOUP

1¼ cups condensed tomato soup
⅔ cup Mull-Soy
⅔ cup water

Blend all ingredients in a saucepan. Cook over low heat to serving temperature. Serve at once. Makes 2½ cups.

Note: Canned condensed soups not containing milk or strained vegetables may be used in place of the condensed tomato soup.

CREAMED FRESH PEA SOUP

½ cup Soyalac (concentrated liquid)
½ cup water
1 (10-ounce) package frozen peas (slightly thawed)
Salt to taste

Liquefy together until very smooth. Add ¼ to ½ cup extra water, if too thick. Salt to taste and heat. Serve at once. Makes 1 cup.

Note: Frozen corn or any other frozen vegetable may be used in place of peas.

Variations: Using Basic Cream Sauce recipe*. For cream soup use 1 cup thin cream sauce plus ½ cup finely chopped or pureed vegetables. Season to taste.

*See recipe under Sauces, this part.

MULL-SOY CREAM SOUP

1 tablespoon vegetable shortening
1½ tablespoons corn-free flour
¼ to ½ teaspoon salt
1 cup Mull-Soy
1 cup water
1 cup cooked, strained or mashed vegetables*

Melt shortening in saucepan over low heat. Remove from heat and blend in flour and salt. Gradually stir in the Mull-Soy, keeping mixture smooth. Stir in water and cook over medium heat, stirring constantly, until thickened. Blend in vegetables. Heat to serving temperature and serve at once. Makes 3 cups.

*Use vegetables such as peas, spinach, asparagus, celery or potatoes that are included in your diet. Liquid drained from cooked vegetables may be used in place of water to enhance the flavor and food value.

BAKED FISH WITH TOMATOES

2 (2½-pound) fish (any kind)
1 pint (2 cup) diced fresh or canned tomatoes
⅓ cup chopped green pepper
Sprinkle of pepper and salt
2 tablespoons olive oil
1 teaspoon cane or beet sugar
Cottonside oil for baking dish

Oil baking dish, lay fish on it. Cover with tomatoes, green pepper. Season with salt, pepper to taste, and sugar. Pour about 1 tablespoon olive oil over all. Bake in hot oven 425°F. until tender, about 20 minutes. Serves 4 to 6.

MULL-SOY VEGETABLE CREAM SOUP

1 (No. 2) can vegetables*
1 tablespoon CORNSTARCH
¼ to ½ teaspoon salt
1 cup Mull-Soy
1 tablespoon soy shortening

Drain vegetables, reserving liquid. Press vegetables through a coarse sieve and set aside. Measure vegetable liquid to make 1½ cups. If not enough, add water. Pour into a 1-quart saucepan. Sprinkle cornstarch and salt on surface of liquid and let stand for a few minutes. Stir until cornstarch is blended. Stir in Mull-Soy and shortening. Bring to a boil, stirring constantly, and boil gently for 5 minutes. Stir in sieved vegetables and reheat to serving temperature. Makes 2½ cups.

*Use vegetables such as peas, green beans and carrots that are included in your diet. Two cups of fresh or frozen vegetables cooked in 2 cups boiling water may be used in place of canned vegetables.

TOMATO SOUP

4 cups peeled tomatoes
2 cups water
2 teaspoons sugar
1 teaspoon salt
4 cloves
1 slice onion (or garlic salt)
⅛ teaspoon baking soda
2 tablespoons BUTTER
2 tablespoons potato flour

Cook the first 6 ingredients for 20 minutes. Strain, reheat and add the soda. In a saucepan, melt the butter, add flour and stir until smooth. Gradually add the hot strained tomato mixture. Serves 4.

POULTRY

CHICKEN SUPRÊME

- **1 (4½- to 5-pound) chicken**
- **4 to 6 cups cooked rice**
- **4 cups chicken broth**
- **4 tablespoons chicken fat**
- **¾ cup rice FLOUR**
- **1 teaspoon salt**
- **3 cups Mull-Soy**
- **1 (2-ounce) can pimientos**
- **1 (6-ounce) can mushrooms**
- **1 cup toasted and shredded almonds**
- **3 tablespoons melted BUTTER**
- **3 tablespoons bread crumbs**

Cook chicken in water, until tender. Cook rice according to directions, then drain. Remove chicken from bones. Pour 1 cup of broth over rice, and set aside. Melt fat in large pan, stir in flour and salt. Add remaining 3 cups broth and Mull-Soy. When thickened add chicken, rice and remaining ingredients. Mix crumbs and melted butter and cover chicken-rice mixture. Bake at 350°F. for 45 minutes. Serves 10 to 12.

CHICKEN BAKED WITH OYSTERS

- **1 (3-pound) chicken**
- **¼ cup rice FLOUR**
- **1½ teaspoons salt**
- **Pinch of pepper**
- **¼ cup salad oil**
- **¼ cup hot water**
- **1 dozen oysters, drained**
- **¾ cup Mull-Soy**

Wash chicken. Dry and quarter. Mix flour with 1 teaspoon salt and pepper. Dredge chicken and brown in oil. Add water, cover and cook slowly for 30 minutes. Place chicken in a shallow baking dish. Add oysters. Mix Mull-Soy and remaining salt, pour into baking dish. Bake in a 350F. oven for 30 minutes. Serves 4.

MEXICANA CHICKEN

1 (3-pound) chicken
3 tablespoons salad oil
1 teaspoon rice FLOUR
1 medium-sized onion, sliced
2½ cups cooked tomatoes
1 teaspoon salt
Pinch of pepper
1 teaspoon chili powder
Hot cooked rice

Wash and dry chicken, then split. Brown chicken in oil in a Dutch oven and remove. Blend flour into the oil. Add the onion, tomatoes, salt, pepper and chili powder. Heat. Add chicken, cover and simmer for 1 hour and 15 minutes. Serve over rice. Serves 4.

POULTRY STUFFINGS

HOECAKE STUFFING (See recipe Part 9)

VEGETABLES

STUFFED POTATOES

6 large baking potatoes
2 tablespoons chicken fat, melted
1 EGG yolk
Salt and pepper to taste

Wash potatoes. Bake until tender. Cut slice off top, remove potato from shells and mash. Add chicken fat seasoning and egg yolk. Refill shells and bake 15 minutes longer. Serve hot. Serves 6.

CREAMED CARROTS

2 cups diced cooked carrots
1 cup Basic Medium Cream Sauce*
2 teaspoons chopped parsley

Mix carrots and cream sauce. Heat thoroughly and garnish with parsley. Serves 2.

Note: Any other desired vegetable may be used in place of carrots.

*See Basic Medium Cream Sauce recipe, this part.

MASHED POTATOES

4 medium-sized potatoes
2 teaspoons soy margarine
1 teaspoon salt
Dash of pepper
2 cups Sobee liquid
2 cups water
Dash of paprika (optional)

Boil potatoes, covered, in salted water until tender, about 20 minutes. Drain and mash. Add margarine, salt, pepper, mixing well. Heat Sobee liquid and water. Add to potatoes and beat until potatoes are light and fluffy.

Note: Add a dash of paprika before serving. Serves 4.

DESSERTS

Cakes

APPLESAUCE CAKE CARLETON

1¾ cups cake FLOUR
1 teaspoon baking powder
½ teaspoon baking soda
½ teaspoon salt
1 teaspoon cinnamon
½ teaspoon cloves
½ cup Crisco
1 cup sugar
1 EGG, well beaten
1 cup raisins, finely cut and FLOURED
1 cup chopped nuts
¾ cup strained, hot thick applesauce

Sift flour once and measure. Add baking powder, soda, salt and spices. Sift together three times. Cream Crisco thoroughly and add sugar gradually. Cream together until light and fluffy. Add egg, raisins and nuts. Add flour mixture alternately with applesauce, a small amount at a time. Beat after each addition until smooth. Bake in greased 8x5x3-inch loaf pan in a 350°F. oven for about 1 hour. Serves 8 to 10.

APPLESAUCE CAKE

1¾ cups sifted corn-free cake flour
1 teaspoon corn-free baking powder
1 teaspoon baking soda
¼ teaspoon salt
1 teaspoon cinnamon
½ teaspoon cloves
½ cup Crisco
1 cup cane, beet or fruit sugar
1 EGG, well beaten
1 cup raisins, finely cut and dusted with corn-free flour
1 cup chopped nuts
¾ cup strained, hot thick applesauce

Sift flour once and measure. Add baking powder, soda, salt and spices. Sift together three times. Cream Crisco thoroughly. Add sugar gradually and cream together until light and fluffy.

Add egg, raisins and nuts. Add flour mixture alternately with applesauce, a small amount at a time. Beat well after each addition until smooth. Bake in greased 8x5x3-inch loaf pan in a 350°F. oven for about 1 hour. Serves 10 to 12.

SWISS CHOCOLATE CAKE

½ cup corn-free margarine
¾ teaspoon salt
1 teaspoon vanilla
1¼ cups cane, beet or fruit sugar
2 EGGS, unbeaten
1 ounce chocolate, melted
2 cups sifted corn-free cake flour
2½ teaspoons corn-free baking powder
1 cup water

Combine margarine, salt and vanilla. Add sugar gradually and cream until light and fluffy. Add eggs, one at a time, beating well after each addition. Blend in melted chocolate. Sift flour and baking powder together three times. Add small amount of flour to margarine mixture alternately with water, beating after each addition until smooth. Grease two 8-inch square layer pans with corn-free margarine. Bake at 350°F. for 30 minutes. Frost. Serves 8 to 10.

CHOCOLATE ROLL

6 tablespoons corn-free cake flour
½ teaspoon corn-free baking powder
¼ teaspoon salt
4 EGGS, separated
¾ cup sifted cane, beet or fruit sugar
1 teaspoon vanilla
4 ounces bitter chocolate, melted
Confectioners' sugar
Mint Frosting (recipe follows)

Sift flour and measure. Add baking powder and salt, sifting together three times. Stiffly beat egg whites and fold in sugar gradually. Beat egg yolks and vanilla. Add yolks to whites. Fold in flour mixture gradually. Gently beat in 2 ounces of the chocolate thoroughly. Turn into 10x15-inch pan which has been greased, lined with paper within ½ inch of edge and again greased. Bake in a 400°F. oven for 13 minutes, or until done.

Cut off crisp edges quickly. Turn out on to a cloth covered with confectioners' sugar and remove paper. Spread half of mint frosting over cake and roll. Wrap in a cloth and cool about 5 minutes. Cover with remaining frosting. When frosting is set, cover with bitter sweet coating made by melting the remaining 2 ounces of chocolate. Serves 6.

MINT FROSTING

2 EGG whites, unbeaten
1½ cups cane, beet or fruit sugar
5 tablespoons water
1½ teaspoons maple syrup
Green coloring
¼ teaspoon peppermint extract

Combine egg whites, sugar, water and maple syrup in the top of a double boiler, beating with rotary eggbeater until thoroughly mixed. Place over rapidly boiling water, beating constantly with egg beater. Cook for 7 minutes, or until frosting will stand in peaks. Add coloring gradually to give a delicate tint. Remove from boiling water, add peppermint extract and beat until thick enough to spread.

MOCHA LAYER CAKE

6 EGGS, separated
1 cup cane, beet or fruit sugar
1 tablespoon mocha essence
1 teaspoon corn-free baking powder
1 cup corn-free flour

Beat egg whites until stiff. Beat egg yolks until thick. Add sugar to yolks and continue beating. Add mocha flavoring and egg whites. Combine baking powder and flour and sift into egg mixture. Pour into two cake pans. Bake in a 350°F. oven for 30 to 40 minutes. Frost with an icing of confectioners' sugar and water blended until smooth and flavored with a few drops of mocha essence. Serves 6 to 8.

DELICATE WHITE LAYER CAKE

2½ cups sifted corn-free cake flour
3 teaspoons corn-free baking powder
¼ teaspoon cream of tartar
½ cup corn-free margarine
1½ cups sifted cane, beet or fruit sugar
½ cup water
1 teaspoon vanilla
6 EGG whites, stiffly beaten
Frosting* (optional)

Sift flour once and measure. Add baking powder and cream of tartar and sift together three times. Cream margarine thoroughly, add sugar gradually and cream together until light and fluffy. Add flour mixture alternately with water, a little at a time. Beat after each addition until smooth. Add vanilla. Fold in egg whites. Pour into two greased 9-inch layer cake pans. Bake in a 375°F. oven for 30 minutes. Serves 10 to 12.

*Ice with any corn- and milk-free frosting, if desired.

JELLY ROLL

¾ cup sifted corn-free cake flour
¼ teaspoon salt
¾ teaspoon corn-free baking powder
4 EGGS, unbeaten
1 scant cup cane, beet or fruit sugar
1 teaspoon vanilla
Confectioners' sugar
1 cup jelly (any kind)

Sift flour once and measure. Combine salt, baking powder and eggs in a bowl. Place over small bowl of hot water and beat with rotary beater, adding sugar gradually until mixture becomes thick and light-colored. Remove bowl from hot water. Fold in flour and vanilla. Turn into a 15x10-inch pan that has been greased, lined with waxed paper to within ½ inch of edge, then greased again. Bake in a 400°F. oven for 13 minutes. Quickly cut off crisp edges of cake. Turn out on cloth covered with confectioners' sugar, removing paper, spread fast with jelly and roll. Wrap in cloth and cool on rack. Serves 4 to 5.

ONE-EGG CAKE

- **1 cup cane, beet or fruit sugar**
- **2 tablespoons peanut oil (or Crisco)**
- **1 EGG, well beaten**
- **Water or coconut milk**
- **2 cups sifted corn-free flour**
- **2 teaspoons corn-free baking powder**
- **½ teaspoon vanilla**

Grease an oblong cake pan or muffin tins. Cream sugar with peanut oil. Put egg in a cup, beat well, and fill cup with water (or coconut milk). Transfer to a bowl, add flour, baking powder and vanilla. Bake in a 400°F. for about 25 minutes. Serves 8.

ORANGE CAKE

- **¾ cup peanut oil or Crisco**
- **1½ cups beet, cane or fruit sugar**
- **3 EGGS, separated**
- **¼ cup strained orange juice**
- **¼ cup water**
- **2¼ cups corn-free flour**
- **3½ teaspoons corn-free baking powder**
- **½ teaspoon salt**
- **1 tablespoon grated orange rind**
- **Orange Filling (recipe follows)**

Cream oil and sugar, then add egg yolks. Beat egg whites until stiff. Sift dry ingredients together. Alternately add orange juice, water and sifted dry ingredients. Add beaten whites, then rind. Bake in a 350°F. oven for 30 to 35 minutes. Serves 10.

ORANGE FILLING

- **1 cup orange juice**
- **1½ teaspoons lemon juice**
- **1 cup cane, beet or fruit sugar**
- **2 tablespoons grated orange rind**
- **½ teaspoon salt**
- **2 tablespoons arrowroot**

Heat juices in the top of a double boiler. Add sugar, orange rind and salt. Thicken with arrowroot and cook for about 15 minutes. When cool, spread between layers. Ice cake with boiled icing.

SPONGE CAKE, NO. 1

Pinch of salt
3 EGGS, separated
3 tablespoons water (or coconut milk)
1 teaspoon baking powder
1 cup corn-free flour
1 cup cane, beet or fruit sugar
⅓ teaspoon vanilla

Combine salt, egg yolks and beat until thick and light. Stiffly beat egg whites. Sift baking powder and flour. Add ½ cup of the sugar to the yolks with vanilla, egg whites and flour. Grease an oblong pan, cover with waxed paper, then grease paper. Bake in a preheated 400°F. oven from 35 to 50 minutes. Serves 6 to 8.

SPONGE CAKE, NO. 2

4 EGGS
1 cup cane, beet or fruit sugar
1 cup corn-free flour
1 teaspoon corn-free baking powder
½ teaspoon vanilla or lemon juice

Separate eggs and beat yolks until very light. Add ½ cup sugar to egg whites and beat until very stiff. Add the remaining ½ cup sugar to egg yolks. Combine yolks and whites and beat hard. Combine flour and baking powder and fold in. Add vanilla or lemon juice. Pour into angel cake pan. Bake in a 300°F. oven for about 40 minutes. Serves 6 to 8.

GINGERBREADS (See recipe Part 9)

CLAUDIA'S CUPCAKES (See recipe Part 9)

RAISIN LOAF (See recipe Part 9)

CHAMPION FRUITCAKE (See recipe Part 9)

PINEAPPLE UPSIDE-DOWN CAKE (See recipe Part 9)

CARROT CAKE

5 EGGS, separated
1 cup cane, beet or fruit sugar
2 tablespoons potato flour
1 teaspoon allspice
1 teaspoon cinnamon
1 teaspoon vanilla
½ cup ground carrots
1 cup chopped nuts
Pinch of salt

Beat the egg whites until stiff. Beat the egg yolks and add the remaining ingredients, the beaten egg whites last. Pour into two layer cake pans. Bake in a preheated 400°F. oven for 40 to 50 minutes. Serves 8 to 10.

RICE CAKES

4 EGG whites, slightly beaten
⅓ cup cane, beet or fruit sugar
1 cup rice FLOUR, sifted twice
1 teaspoon vanilla
½ cup soy BUTTER, softened

Beat egg whites slightly. Add sugar and flour, stirring it in very lightly. Add vanilla and butter. Drop by tablespoonfuls on greased cookie sheet 2 to 3 inches apart. Using the back of a floured spoon, spread thin. Bake in 325°F. oven for 10 minutes. They will be thin and crisp. Makes about 2 dozen.

*SPONGE CAKE, NO. 3

4 EGGS, separated
4 tablespoons granulated cane, beet or fruit sugar
1 level teaspoon corn-free baking powder
5 tablespoons potato flour
Vanilla

Stiffly beat egg whites and add sugar. Add yolks and remaining ingredients. Pour into a 10x15-inch pan with a greased waxed paper lining. Bake at 320°F. for 40 minutes.

SPONGE CAKE JELLY ROLL

Potato flour sponge cake* baked in a 10x15-inch pan. Spread with any kind of jelly. Roll and dust with powdered cane, beet or fruit sugar.

CAROB BROWNIES, NO. 1

½ cup vegetable oil
¼ cup honey
2 EGGS
1 teaspoon vanilla
½ teaspoon salt
3 tablespoons water
⅔ cup wheat FLOUR
⅓ cup carob powder
1 teaspoon baking powder
½ cup chopped nuts

Cream oil and honey. Beat in eggs, vanilla and salt. Sift flour, carob and baking powder. Add with water to other ingredients; blend well. Stir in nuts. Pour into an 8x8x2-inch greased pan. Bake in a 325°F. oven 20 to 25 minutes. Makes about 1 dozen.

CAROB ROLL

6 EGGS, separated
1 cup granulated cane, beet or fruit sugar
1 cup carob powder
Mint jelly
Confectioners' sugar

Stiffly beat egg whites. Cream yolks and granulated sugar together. Add carob and egg whites. Grease waxed paper on both sides with chicken fat or some cottonseed product. Line an oblong pan and pour in batter. Bake in a preheated 275°F. oven for about 15 minutes. Cover with mint jelly. Roll when cold. Sprinkle with confectioners' sugar. Serves 4 to 6.

CAROB BROWNIES, NO. 2

2 EGGS
¼ cup sifted rice or rye FLOUR
1 teaspoon vanilla
1¼ cups cane, beet or fruit sugar
½ cup chopped nuts
½ cup carob powder

Beat eggs slightly. Stir in remaining ingredients. Spread batter evenly in an 8x8x2-inch greased pan. Bake at 375°F. for 20 minutes. Cut when cooled. Makes about 2½ dozen.

NUT AND BUTTER CAKE

½ cup barley flour
½ cup rye FLOUR
½ cup potato flour
Pinch of salt
1 teaspoon corn-free baking powder
1 cup corn-free margarine
1 cup cane, beet or fruit sugar
2 EGGS, separated
6 tablespoons Soyamel
½ cup chopped nuts
1 teaspoon vanilla

Sift flours with salt and baking powder. Cream margarine and sugar. Beat egg yolks and add to sugar, mixing until creamy. Add the Soyamel and flour mixture alternately, beating well. Add nuts and vanilla. Stiffly beat egg whites and fold in. Pour into a greased baking pan. Bake at 350°F. for 25 to 30 minutes. Serves 8.

SPICE CAKE WITH PINEAPPLE ICING (See recipe Part 11)

PINEAPPLE ICING (See recipe Part 11)

WHITE CAKE WITH SOY FLOUR (See recipe Part 11)

SPICY SUGAR CAKE (See recipe Part 11)

MARBLE CAKE

1½ tablespoons corn-free margarine
3 tablespoons cane, beet or fruit sugar
4 tablespoons cocoa
3 tablespoons water
1 cup cane, beet or fruit sugar
½ cup corn free margarine
½ teaspoon salt
1 teaspoon vanilla
2 EGGS, unbeaten
2 cups sifted corn-free cake flour
2½ teaspoons corn-free baking powder
⅔ cup water

Cook first four ingredients until smooth, then cool. Cream 1 cup sugar, ½ cup margarine, salt and vanilla. Add eggs, one at a time, beating thoroughly after each addition. Sift flour and baking powder together. Add to sugar mixture, a little at a time, alternating with water. Beat until smooth. Divide batter into two parts. Add cocoa mixture to one half. Place chocolate and white batters alternately, a tablespoon at a time to form a black/white look, in an 8x8x2-inch pan greased with margarine. Bake in a 350°F. oven for 60 minutes. Serves 8.

MATZO MEAL CAKE

8 EGGS, separated
1½ cups cane, beet or fruit sugar
⅛ teaspoon salt
Juice and grated rind of ½ lemon (or 1 teaspoon vanilla)
1 cup finely sifted matzo meal
Lord Baltimore Frosting*

Beat egg yolks until lemon colored. Beat in sugar and salt. Add lemon and matzo meal. Stiffly beat egg whites and fold in. Pour batter into a springform pan or in two layer pans. Bake in a preheated 400°F. oven for 35 to 50 minutes. Ice with Lord Baltimore Frosting. Serves 8 to 10.

*See following recipe.

LORD BALTIMORE FROSTING

- **¾ cup cane or beet sugar**
- **1 EGG white, beaten stiff**
- **Pinch of corn-free baking powder**
- **½ teaspoon flavoring**
- **½ cup rolled macaroon crumbs***
- **¼ cup water**
- **½ cup chopped pecans**
- **2 teaspoons sherry**
- **½ teaspoon lemon juice**

Boil sugar and water to long-threads stage. Pour in a fine stream over the beaten egg whites until mixture thickens. Add baking powder and flavoring and add macaroon crumbs, chopped pecans, sherry, and lemon juice. Spread. Makes about 2¼ cups.

*See recipe for Almond Macaroons, Part 15.

ORANGE LAYER CAKE

- **2 cups cane, beet or fruit sugar**
- **5 EGG yolks**
- **Juice and grated rind of 1 orange**
- **½ cup water or coconut milk**
- **2 cups corn-free flour**
- **1 teaspoon corn-free baking powder**
- **3 EGG whites, stiffly beaten for cake (save 2 for icing)**
- **Icing***

Cream sugar and egg yolks. Add orange juice, water, part of the rind (save rest for icing) and flour (sifted 3 times with baking powder). Fold in egg whites. Grease an oblong pan, line with waxed paper and grease again. Pour mixture into pan. Bake in a preheated 375°F. oven for 40 minutes. Serves 8 to 10.

*Icing recipe follows.

ICING

Two stiffly beaten EGG whites
1 cup confectioners' sugar
1 teaspoon grated orange rind

Spread over cake.

MOCHA AND RAISIN NUT BARS

1 package white cake mix (check label)
1 cup cold coffee
2 EGGS
1 cup chopped raisins
1 cup chopped nuts

Empty cake mix into bowl and add coffee and eggs. Beat until smooth and creamy, about 3 minutes. Add raisins and nuts, mixing well. Pour into 2 greased 9x13-inch pans. Bake at 350°F. for about 25 minutes, or until a straw inserted in center comes out clean. Cool. Makes 5 dozen.

Ice Cream

ICE CREAM

In making ICE CREAM, the best method to use is the regular old-fashioned ICE CREAM freezer (electric or hand-operated). This makes the smoothest ICE CREAM. The following recipe will be creamy and have a fine texture, if made in this way. It may also be made in the freezing compartment of the refrigerator, but should be whipped once or twice while freezing.

VANILLA ICE CREAM

¼ cup CORN OIL
⅛ teaspoon salt
1 cup Soyalac powder
½ cup honey (clover is mild tasting)
2½ cups water
1 tablespoon vanilla

Place all ingredients in liquefier and blend. Freeze in hand freezer. This can be varied by adding fruit, nuts and different flavors. Makes 1 quart.

Note: 3½ cups Soyalac concentrated liquid may be used in place of the Soyalac powder and water.

Candy

SOYALAC CAROB FUDGE

2 cups white or brown cane, beet or fruit sugar
2 tablespoons carob powder
¼ cup CORN SYRUP
¼ cup Soyalac (concentrated liquid)
¼ cup water
2 tablespoons corn-free margarine
1 teaspoon vanilla

Combine first five ingredients. Cook until mixture forms a soft ball in cold water or registers 230°F. on candy thermometer. Stir frequently while cooking. Remove from heat, cool slightly and add margarine and vanilla. Beat until thick. Pour onto an oiled plate. Refrigerate until hardened.

Note: Chocolate may be substituted, if desired.

Cookies

CHOCOLATE SQUARES

- **⅓ cup peanut or cottonseed oil**
- **1 cup cane, beet or fruit sugar**
- **2 EGGS**
- **2 ounces chocolate, melted**
- **¾ cup corn-free cake flour**
- **½ teaspoon salt**
- **1 cup chopped nuts**
- **1 teaspoon vanilla**

Cream oil and sugar thoroughly. Add remaining ingredients. Pour into a greased 8-inch square shallow pan. Bake at 325°F. for 20 minutes. Cut into squares before removing from pan. Makes 2 dozen.

DATE-COCONUT MACAROONS (See recipe Part 9)

MOLASSES COOKIES (See recipe Part 9)

*ALMOND MACAROONS (See recipe Part 15)

DATE PECAN PUFFS (See recipe Part 15)

TEA WAFERS (See recipe Part 15)

DATE AND WALNUT DROPS (See recipe Part 15)

OATMEAL COOKIES, NO. 1 (See recipe Part 11)

OATMEAL COOKIES, NO. 2 (See recipe Part 11)

SOYALAC NUT CRESCENTS (See recipe Part 11)

CHOCOLATE POTATO DROP CAKES

- **1 cup cane, beet or fruit sugar**
- **½ cup peanut or cottonseed oil or soy margarine**
- **2 EGGS, separated**
- **2 ounces chocolate, grated**
- **1 cup mashed potatoes**
- **⅓ cup raisins**
- **1 cup wheat FLOUR**
- **1 level tablespoon corn-free baking powder**
- **½ teaspoon salt**
- **Chopped nuts (optional)**

Cream sugar and oil or fat. Beat in egg yolks. Add chocolate, potatoes and raisins. Add flour sifted with the baking powder and salt. Stiffly beat egg whites and fold in. Drop by tablespoonfuls onto greased cookie sheets. Bake in a 375°F. oven for 20 to 25 minutes. Makes about 2 dozen.

Note: Chopped nuts may be added.

HICKORY NUT COOKIES

- **3 EGGS**
- **⅓ cup cane, beet or fruit sugar**
- **¾ chopped hickory nuts**
- **⅓ cup soy shortening, melted**
- **1½ cups corn-free flour**
- **½ cup brown cane, beet or fruit sugar**
- **½ teaspoon salt**
- **¼ teaspoon corn-free baking powder**
- **¼ teaspoon baking soda**
- **½ teaspoon vanilla**

Beat eggs, sugar, nuts and shortening together. Sift dry ingredients, and add to egg mixture. Add vanilla. Drop by teaspoonfuls far apart on greased baking sheet. Bake in a 350°F. oven for 12 to 15 minutes. Makes 4 dozen.

KEWPIES

1 cup soy margarine
1½ cups brown cane, beet or fruit sugar
3 EGGS, beaten
3 cups corn-free flour
1 level teaspoon baking soda
2 cups chopped nuts
1 pound raisins

Mix all ingredients together into a stiff batter. Drop by teaspoons onto a warm greased pan. Bake at 400°F. for about 10 minutes. Makes 4 dozen.

Puddings

CLARET MACAROON PUDDING

1½ dozen small almond macaroons
Dash of cinnamon (optional)
1 cup granulated cane, beet or fruit sugar
1 tablespoon CORNSTARCH
3 EGGS, separated
1½ cups claret
⅛ cup confectioners' sugar
⅛ teaspoon lemon juice
⅔ cup blanched almonds

Break macaroons into quarters and arrange on an oven platter. Mix cinnamon, granulated sugar and cornstarch. Add to beaten yolks, then slowly mix in claret. Heat in the top of a double boiler, stirring constantly, until mixture coats the spoon. Pour, while hot, over macaroons.

Cover with meringue made as follows: Beat egg whites until foamy. Gradually add confectioners' sugar and continue beating until mixture stands in peaks. Add lemon juice. Spread on pudding and dot with almonds. Bake in a 350°F. oven for 15 minutes, or until lightly browned. Serve hot or cold. Serves 8.

SOYALAC WHIP (See recipe Part 9)

FROZEN MULL-SOY DELIGHT

1 cup Mull-Soy
3 tablespoons cane, beet or fruit sugar
1 teaspoon unflavored gelatin
1 tablespoon water
1 teaspoon vanilla

Chill Mull-Soy. Add sugar and beat with rotary beater or electric mixer until sugar is dissolved. Soften gelatin in water for 3 minutes. Place over hot water, stirring until gelatin is dissolved. Stir into Mull-Soy mixture with vanilla. Pour into freezing tray. Cover tray with waxed paper and freeze to a firm mush. Remove waxed paper and pour into chilled bowl. Beat with rotary beater or electric mixer until fluffy but not melted. Quickly return to freezing tray and return to freezing unit. Freeze until firm. Makes about 2 cups.

CAROB PUDDING

2 tablespoons CORNSTARCH
5 tablespoons brown cane, beet or fruit sugar
2 tablespoons carob powder
Pinch of salt
⅔ cup Soyalac (liquid)
⅔ cup water
1 teaspoon vanilla

Combine dry ingredients in top of double boiler. Gradually add Soyalac and water, which have been mixed together. Cook over boiling water, stirring constantly, until thickened and smooth. Cover and cook for 15 minutes, stirring occasionally. Remove from heat and add vanilla. Serve cold. Serves 2.

Note: Chocolate may be substituted, if permitted.

CORNSTARCH PUDDING

2 tablespoons CORNSTARCH
¼ cup cane, beet or fruit sugar
Pinch of salt
¾ cup Mull-Soy
¾ cup water
½ teaspoon vanilla

Combine cornstarch, sugar and salt in the top of a double boiler. Gradually stir in Mull-Soy, keeping mixture smooth. Stir in water. Cook over boiling water, stirring constantly, until thickened and smooth, about 5 minutes. Cover and cook for 15 minutes, stirring occasionally. Remove from heat and stir in vanilla. Turn into serving dishes and chill. Serves 3.

Variations:
Coffee: Use ¾ cup strong coffee beverage in place of water.
Chocolate: Add 1½ ounces unsweetened chocolate, cut in small pieces, to the cornstarch-sugar mixture and increase the sugar to 5 tablespoons.

PINEAPPLE DESSERT

½ envelope gelatin
¼ cup cold water
½ cup Nutramigen beverage
3 tablespoons cane, beet or fruit sugar
Dash of salt
2 tablespoons lemon juice
Few drops yellow food coloring
2 tablespoons drained, crushed pineapple

Sprinkle gelatin on water and let set for 1 minute. Heat Nutramigen, sugar, salt and lemon juice to lukewarm. Add gelatin and stir until dissolved. Add food color and pineapple, mix well and chill. Serves 1 to 2.

INDIAN PUDDING

- **¼ cup yellow CORNMEAL**
- **¼ cup water**
- **1 cup Mull-Soy**
- **1 cup boiling water**
- **½ cup raisins or finely diced prunes**
- **½ cup molasses**

Combine cornmeal and ¼ cup water in top of double boiler. Let stand 5 minutes. Stir in Mull-Soy and then the boiling water. Cook over boiling water, stirring often, until thickened, about 20 minutes. Mix in raisins or chopped prunes and molasses. Pour into a greased 1-quart casserole or baking dish. Bake in a 325°F. oven for 2 hours. Serve hot. Serves 4 to 6.

Torte

DATE TORTE

- **4 EGGS**
- **1 cup cane, beet or fruit sugar**
- **¼ cup cracker crumbs**
- **1 teaspoon corn-free baking powder**
- **½ cup chopped walnuts**
- **1 cup chopped pitted dates**
- **Sherry**

Separate eggs and beat yolks. Add sugar gradually, then cracker crumbs, baking powder, nuts and dates. Stiffly beat egg whites and fold in. Bake 1 hour or longer in a 300°F. oven. Cut into squares. To serve, pour sherry over cake. Makes about 2 dozen.

SAUCES

BROWN SAUCE

1½ tablespoons fat
2 tablespoons FLOUR
1 teaspoon onion juice or garlic salt
1 cup meat stock or hot water
Salt and pepper

Brown fat with flour and onion juice (if allergic to onions, season with a very few grains of garlic salt). Add meat stock. Cook until thick and smooth. Season to taste with salt and pepper. Makes 1¼ cups.

WHITE SAUCE MADE WITH GOAT'S MILK

1 tablespoon chicken fat
1 tablespoon corn-free flour
½ cup goat's MILK
½ cup cold water
Salt

Melt fat and stir in flour, mixing well. Add goat's milk, which has been mixed with cold water. Cook, stirring, until thickened. Season with a little salt. Makes about 1 cup.

Note: Goat's milk is used here as a substitute for cow's milk but does not contain the same casein fraction.

MEDIUM CREAM SAUCE WITH RICE FLOUR

2 tablespoons soy margarine
2 tablespoons rice FLOUR
¾ cup Sobee liquid
½ cup water
Salt and pepper

Melt margarine in a 1-quart saucepan. Add flour, stirring until smooth. Add Sobee liquid and water and cook, stirring constantly, until smooth and thick. Add salt and pepper to taste. Makes about 1½ cups.

RYE FLOUR GRAVY

3 tablespoons corn-free fat drippings
2 tablespoons rye FLOUR
¾ cup Sobee liquid and water, mixed half and half
Salt and pepper to taste

Heat fat in frying pan. Add flour and brown, stirring. Add the Sobee and water mixture slowly, stirring constantly to keep smooth. Cook on low heat until thick and smooth. Add salt and pepper to taste. Makes 1 cup.

MUSHROOM SAUCE
(*Meat*)

1 cup mushrooms
1 cup mushroom liquor
1 level teaspoon CORNSTARCH
1 teaspoon Worcestershire sauce
2 teaspoons catsup
Pinch of salt

Boil mushrooms for 15 minutes. Heat liquor to boiling point. Add cornstarch, which has been thinned with a little cold water, and bring to a boil. Add Worcestershire sauce, catsup and salt. Add mushrooms, which have been cut in half, and simmer for 15 minutes. Makes 2 cups.

BROWN SAUCE WITH MUSHROOMS

2 cups mushrooms
1 teaspoon chopped parsley
1½ tablespoons chicken fat
1 teaspoon onion juice
2 tablespoons FLOUR
1 cup meat stock or hot mushroom water
Salt and pepper

Sauté mushrooms, chop fine and add with parsley to browned chicken fat (or other fat not a dairy product), onion juice, and flour. Add meat stock. Cook until smooth and thick. Season with a little salt and pepper. Makes approximately 3 cups.

BASIC CREAM SAUCE

	Thin	Medium	Thick
Vegetable margarine or oil, Chicken, beef, bacon or lamb drippings	1 tablespoon	1 tablespoon	2 tablespoons
Thickening agent (use only one)			
wheat FLOUR	1 tablespoon	2 tablespoons	3 tablespoons
rye FLOUR	2 tablespoons	3 tablespoons	4 tablespoons
cornstarch	1 tablespoon	2 tablespoons	3 tablespoons
arrowroot flour	2 teaspoons	1½ tablespoons	2 tablespoons
rice FLOUR	2 teaspoons	1½ tablespoons	2 tablespoons
Salt	¼ teaspoon	¼ teaspoon	½ teaspoon
Mull-Soy or Soyalac (concentrated liquid)	½ cup	½ cup	½ cup
Water	½ cup	½ cup	½ cup

Blend fat, thickening agent and salt. Add Mull-Soy or Soyalac and water. Cook over low heat, stirring constantly, until thick and thoroughly cooked. Use thin cream sauce for soups, medium for scalloped or creamed dishes and thick for croquettes.

LEMON SAUCE

2 tablespoons lemon juice
½ cup water
½ cup sugar
Grated rind of 1 lemon
1½ tablespoons CORNSTARCH
¼ cup cold water
1 EGG yolk

Cook first four ingredients. Add cornstarch, which has been blended in cold water. When mixture has thickened remove from heat, add egg yolk and beat. Serve cold. Makes approximately 1½ cups.

PINEAPPLE SAUCE

1 tablespoon CORNSTARCH
½ cup pineapple juice
1 cup crushed pineapple
⅛ cup sugar

Blend cornstarch and pineapple juice. Add remaining ingredients and cook, stirring constantly. Serve with ice cream or tapioca. Makes approximately 1½ cups.

GINGERSNAP SAUCE

4 gingersnaps
¼ cup brown sugar
¼ cup vinegar
½ teaspoon onion juice
1 cup hot water
1 lemon, sliced
¼ cup raisins
Soup or fish stock

Combine all ingredients and cook until smooth. Serve hot or cold with fish, meat, tongue or leftover meat. Makes approximately 1½ cups.

BEVERAGES

CAROB-COCONUT SHAKE

½ cup Soyalac (concentrate)
½ teaspoon carob powder
¼ cup water
2 teaspoons coconut syrup

Mix all ingredients together until well blended. Chill before serving. Makes about 1 cup.

SOYALAC TROPICAL DRINK

½ cup Soyalac (concentrate)
1 tablespoon berry concentrate (boysenberry punch or other berry or fruit punch)
½ cup pineapple juice
½ banana
½ cup water

Liquefy all together. Chill and serve. Banana may be mashed and whipped into the other ingredients. Makes 1½ cups.

COFFEE DRINK

¼ cup Mull-Soy
¾ cup strong coffee*
2 tablespoons cane, beet or fruit sugar
Ice cubes (optional)

Combine Mull-Soy, coffee and sugar. If a hot beverage is desired, heat mixture to serving temperature. If a chilled beverage is desired, pour mixture into ice-filled glasses. Makes 1 cup.

*When using instant coffee, dissolve 1½ teaspoons in ¾ cup hot water.

BANANA-PINEAPPLE SHAKE

1 can water
1 can Soyalac (concentrate)
2 small slices pineapple
1 medium-sized banana

Combine water and Soyalac in electric blender. Add pineapple and banana, which has been cut into small pieces. Blend for 1 minute. (More or less fruit may be added according to taste.) Serves 3 to 4.

Note: For one serving use ½ cup Soyalac and ½ cup water with 1 small slice pineapple and ½ banana.

SOYALAC FIG DRINK

½ cup Soyalac
¼ cup water
¼ cup Loma Linda fig juice (or Loma Linda prune juice)

Mix thoroughly and serve hot or cold. This makes a thick beverage that can be thinned with ¼ cup water, if desired. Makes 1 cup.

CREAMY SOBEE LIQUID

1 cup Sobee liquid
½ cup water

Mix well and chill. Makes 1½ cups.

ORANGE BEVERAGE

6 ounces Nutramigen beverage
3 ounces frozen orange juice concentrate

Combine and chill. Serves 1.

LEMON BEVERAGE

8 ounces Nutramigen beverage
3 tablespoons frozen lemon juice
2 tablespoons sugar

Combine and chill. Serves 1.

APRICOT DREAM

½ cup Sobee liquid
½ cup apricot nectar

Mix well and chill. Makes 1 cup.

BANANA SHAKE

1 small, ripe banana
2 tablespoons sugar
½ cup Mull-Soy
½ cup cold water
Pinch of salt
Finely cracked ice

Peel and slice banana. Beat with a rotary or electric beater or in electric blender until smooth and creamy. Beat in sugar. Add Mull-Soy, water and salt and beat until well-blended. Pour into ice-filled glasses and serve at once. Makes 1½ cups.

Note: If allowed, add 2 teaspoons lemon juice with sugar to enhance the flavor.

HAWAIIAN FLING

½ cup Sobee
½ cup pineapple juice
1 teaspoon cane, beet or fruit sugar

Mix well and chill. Makes 1 cup.

SOBEE LIQUID MOCHA

½ cup Sobee liquid
½ cup strong coffee and cocoa mixed

Mix well and chill. Makes 1 cup.

APRICOT MULL-SOY SHAKE

¼ cup Mull-Soy
¼ cup cold water
1 teaspoon lemon juice
½ cup finely cracked ice
½ cup sieved, stewed apricots, sweetened with cane, beet or fruit sugar

Combine all ingredients in a shaker or jar with a tight-fitting lid. Cover container and shake well. Serve at once. Makes approximately 1½ cups.

LEMON DRINK

½ cup Nutramigen beverage
3 rounded teaspoons any powdered commercial lemon drink

Combine and chill. Makes 1 serving.

TANGY DRINK

1 cup Nutramigen beverage
2 teaspoons sugar
3 teaspoons commercial orange powder

Combine and chill. Makes 1 serving.

BANANA-HONEY FLIP

1 cup Sobee liquid
1 ripe banana
1 tablespoon honey

Mix in a blender or mash well with a fork and stir. Makes 1½ cups.

PINEAPPLE FLIP

¼ cup Mull-Soy
¼ cup cold water
1 tablespoon lemon juice
⅓ cup pineapple juice
1 tablespoon cane, beet or fruit sugar
½ cup cracked ice

Combine all ingredients in a shaker or jar with a tight-fitting lid. Cover container and shake well. Serve at once. Makes 1 cup.

PART 14

No Milk, No Wheat

BREADS

QUICK-RAISED RICE BREAD (See recipe Part 13)

COCONUT PANCAKES (See recipe Part 13)

CORNMEAL AND POTATO STARCH MUFFINS

⅔ cup CORNMEAL
2 teaspoons baking powder
½ teaspoon salt
½ teaspoon sugar
⅓ cup potato starch
1 EGG
½ cup water
1 teaspoon fat, melted.

Sift together dry ingredients. Beat egg slightly and add water. Stir gently into dry ingredients. Add fat. Bake in greased muffin tins at 400°F. for 30 minutes. Makes 10 to 12.

SOYBEAN MUFFINS

1 EGG
1 level teaspoon salt
1 tablespoon shortening, melted
2 level teaspoons baking powder
1 tablespoon CORN-STARCH
1¼ cups soybean FLOUR
1 cup water

Beat egg. Stir in salt and shortening. Sift baking powder, cornstarch and flour. Add alternately with water. Fill muffin pans two-thirds full. Bake in a 425°F. to 450°F. oven for 30 to 35 minutes. Makes 1 dozen.

SOYBEAN BREAD

¼ cup CORNSTARCH
¾ cup soybean FLOUR
1 teaspoon salt
2 teaspoons baking powder
1 tablespoon shortening
⅔ cup water
4 EGG yolks
4 EGG whites, stiffly beaten

Sift dry ingredients; add remaining ingredients. Pour into greased loaf tin. Bake in a preheated 400°F. oven for 40 to 50 minutes. Makes 1 loaf.

SOYA CAROB BREAD

1 cake yeast
1¾ cups lukewarm water
4 cups Sterling Soya carob flour
1 tablespoon corn-free sugar or honey
1½ teaspoons salt
2 tablespoons corn-free shortening, melted (or corn-free oil)

Dissolve yeast in lukewarm water. Add remaining ingredients and mix well. Place on a floured board and knead well. Place in large bowl and cover. Let rise in warm place (about 80°F.) until doubled in bulk. Knead down and form into loaves. Place in greased bread pans, grease top of loaf with melted shortening. Let rise until doubled in bulk. Bake in 375°F. oven for about 40 minutes, or until done. Makes 1 large or 2 medium-sized loaves.

SWEET POTATO BREAD

1 cup mashed sweet potatoes
1 cup dry rolled oats and dry CORNMEAL, combined
¾ cup hot water
¾ cup seedless raisins
½ cup chopped walnuts
1 teaspoon salt
3 tablespoons shortening, melted
2 tablespoons honey
1 tablespoon baking powder

Combine potatoes, oats-cornmeal, water and raisins. Add walnuts, salt, shortening, honey and baking powder. Bake in well-greased muffin pans at 400°F. for 20 minutes. Makes 2 dozen.

JOHNNYCAKE

1½ cups CORNMEAL
1½ cups boiling water
¼ cup vegetable shortening, melted
3 teaspoons baking powder
1 teaspoon salt
2 EGGS, separated
¼ cup sugar

Sift cornmeal gradually into boiling water. Remove from heat and add shortening, baking powder, salt and egg yolks. Beat egg whites until stiff, then add sugar and beat until smooth. Fold lightly into cornmeal mixture. Turn immediately into a buttered baking dish, 8 inches square, that has been heated. Bake in a preheated 400°F. oven for 35 minutes, or until golden brown. Serves 4.

BALLS FOR SOUP (See recipe under Breads, Part 15)

RYE AND CORNSTARCH NOODLES

1 EGG
¼ teaspoon salt
¼ cup CORNSTARCH
¼ cup rye FLOUR

Break egg into bowl and add salt. Sift cornstarch and flour together. Add to egg. Refrigerate for 30 minutes. Sift additional cornstarch onto a board. Roll dough very thin. Allow to dry for 15 minutes. Fold in three parts and slice very thin. Set aside to dry for several hours. Drop into boiling soup and cook for 15 minutes. Makes approximately 6 dozen noodles.

SOUPS

SOUP STOCK

2½ pounds beef (plate or brisket)
3 quarts cold water
½ cup raw or stewed tomatoes
¼ cup each onion, carrot, celery, cut up and mixed
1 tablespoon salt
¼ teaspoon pepper
1 teaspoon chopped parsley
Seasoning
Horseradish Sauce*

Wipe and salt meat. Place in soup kettle and let stand 1 hour. Add water and let stand ½ hour longer. Place on stove and bring to a boil. Skim. Let soup simmer 3 hours or more. Add vegetables and cook 1 hour longer, adding more hot water, if necessary. Strain. Cool and skim off fat. Add seasonings. Reheat and add parsley just before serving. Serve soup meat with horseradish sauce. Makes about 2 quarts.

*See recipe under Sauces, this part.

MULLIGATAWNY SOUP

¼ cup sliced onion (optional)
¼ cup diced celery
¼ cup diced carrot
1 teaspoon chopped parsley
1 cup tomato puree
½ green pepper, seeded chopped fine
3 pounds cut-up chicken
4 quarts cold water
2 sour apples, sliced
¼ cup chicken fat
1 tablespoon CORN-STARCH
1 teaspoon curry powder (optional)
2 cloves (optional)
1 teaspoon sugar
1 teaspoon salt
⅛ teaspoon mace (optional)
Pinch of pepper (optional)

Cook vegetables and chicken in fat until brown. Add cornstarch, curry powder, cloves, sugar and all the rest of the ingredients. Cook slowly until the chicken is tender. Remove chicken and cut the meat into small pieces. Strain the soup and rub the vegetables through a sieve. Add the chicken to the strained soup. Season and serve hot with boiled rice. Makes about 5 quarts.

Note: If allergic to spices the optional ingredients may be omitted.

MULL-SOY CREAM SOUP (See recipe Part 13)

CREAMED FRESH PEA SOUP (See recipe Part 13)

TOMATO CREAM SOUP (See recipe Part 13)

MULL-SOY VEGETABLE CREAM SOUP (See recipe Part 13)

TOMATO SOUP (See recipe Part 13)

TOMATO SOUP

2 cups water
4 cloves (optional)
1 slice onion (optional)
2 teaspoons sugar
1 teaspoon salt
⅛ teaspoon baking soda
2 tablespoons chicken fat
2 tablespoons CORNSTARCH
1 quart canned tomatoes

Cook first six ingredients for 20 minutes, then strain. Reheat and add soda. Melt chicken fat; add cornstarch (thinned with a bit of water) and gradually the hot strained tomatoes. Makes about 1½ quarts.

FISH

TUNA CASSEROLE

¾ cup water
¾ cup Sobee liquid
2 tablespoons CORNSTARCH
2 teaspoons minced onion
½ teaspoon celery salt
Dash of garlic salt
1 (6.5-ounce) can tuna, broken into pieces
⅔ cup peas, canned or fresh
2 cups lightly crushed potato chips (save some for top of casserole)

Heat water to boiling. Add Sobee liquid and cornstarch, stirring constantly. Continue stirring until thickened (if sauce seems too thick, add a little more water). Remove sauce from heat and add onion, celery salt, garlic salt and tuna. Lightly stir in peas and potato chips. Pour into greased baking dish and garnish with potato chips. Bake on center rack of a 375°F. to 400°F. oven for 30 to 40 minutes, or until bubbly and brown on top. Serves 4.

POULTRY

CREAMED CHICKEN

- **1 tablespoon chicken fat**
- **1 tablespoon CORN-STARCH**
- **1½ cups diced cooked chicken**
- **1 cup soup stock**
- **1 cup diced cooked celery**
- **3 hard-cooked EGGS, diced**
- **½ can pimiento, cut into strips**
- **Salt**
- **Pepper or paprika**

Blend fat and cornstarch. Add remaining ingredients and heat through. Serves 3 or 4.

CHICKEN SUPRÊME (See recipe Part 13)

POULTRY STUFFING

HOECAKE STUFFING (See recipe Part 9)

VEGETABLES

FRIED EGGPLANT

- **1 large eggplant**
- **Salt**
- **Fat**
- **CORNMEAL or CORNFLAKES**
- **EGGS**

Peel eggplant and slice thinly. Sprinkle with salt. Pile on a plate, cover with weight to extract the juice and let stand for 1½ hours, or soak in brine. Dredge with crushed cornflakes and fry slowly until crisp and brown (or dip in eggs and cornmeal). Serves 4.

DESSERTS

Cakes

COCONUT CAKE

- **1 can coconut**
- **½ cup plus 1 tablespoon sugar**
- **5 EGG yolks**
- **2 tablespoons baking powder**
- **½ cup rye FLOUR**
- **3 heaping teaspoons CORNSTARCH**
- **1 tablespoon cold water**
- **custard (recipe follows)**

Separate coconut milk and meat. Refrigerate ¾ cup of the milk. Cream meat with ½ cup sugar and 4 egg yolks, beating. Stir in ¼ cup cold coconut milk. Blend dry ingredients, and add to coconut mixture. Pour into two greased cake pans (use chicken fat). Bake in a preheated 400° F. oven for 30 minutes. Serves 6.

CUSTARD

Make custard of 1 tablespoon sugar, ½ cup coconut milk and 1 teaspoon cornstarch, blended with 1 tablespoon cold water, and 1 egg yolk. Place custard between half layers. Cover with boiled icing, using 1 egg white.

NUT AND BUTTER CAKE (see recipe Part 13)

CAROB ROLL (See recipe Part 13)

Cookies

ALMOND MACAROONS (See recipe Part 15)

DATE PECAN PUFFS (See recipe Part 15)

TEA WAFERS (See recipe Part 15)

DATE AND WALNUT DROPS (See recipe Part 15)

OATMEAL COOKIES, NO. 1 (See recipe Part 11)

OATMEAL COOKIES, NO. 2 (See recipe Part 11)

SOYALAC NUT CRESCENTS (See recipe Part 11)

CINNAMON STICKS

4 EGG whites
1 pound confectioners' sugar
1 tablespoon cinnamon
2 tablespoons potato flour
Citron, cut up
½ pound almonds, grated

Beat egg whites to a stiff froth. Gradually add sugar, cinnamon, flour, citron and almonds. Dust hands with potato flour. Take 1 teaspoon dough and roll into half finger lengths as thick as one's little finger. Place on greased sheet 1 inch apart. Bake in 300°F. oven for 20 to 30 minutes. Makes approximately 5 dozen.

COCONUT MACAROONS

2 EGGS, whites stiffly beaten
1 cup sugar
¾ cup coconut
2¼ cups CORNFLAKES, crushed
Vanilla

Mix ingredients in order given. Drop by tablespoonfuls on greased cookie sheets. Bake in a 250°F. oven for 25 minutes Makes approximately 2 to 3 dozen.

BILL'S DATE COOKIES

- **1 EGG**
- **¾ cup brown sugar**
- **¼ teaspoon baking powder**
- **⅖ cup oat flour**
- **⅖ cup soybean FLOUR**
- **¼ teaspoon baking soda**
- **¼ cup chopped nuts**
- **¼ cup chopped dates**
- **½ teaspoon vanilla**
- **Vegetable shortening**

Cream egg and sugar. Sift flours together and add to egg mixture. Add remaining ingredients. Drop by teaspoonfuls onto a greased cookie sheet, about 1 inch apart. Bake in a preheated 450°F. oven for about 8 to 12 minutes per pan. Makes 2 dozen.

SHREWSBURY WAFERS

- **3 EGGS**
- **2 cups sugar**
- **2 tablespoons soy shortening, melted**
- **¾ teaspoon vanilla**
- **1 teaspoon salt**
- **1 cup shredded coconut**
- **2 cups rolled oats**

Beat eggs thoroughly. Add sugar gradually, beating constantly. Add shortening, vanilla and salt. Remove beater and stir in coconut and oats. Line shallow pans with greased waxed paper. Drop mixture on this by ½ teaspoonfuls, 1 inch apart. Bake light brown in a preheated 400°F. oven. Lift sheets of paper out of pan, cool partly, then remove. Makes approximately 2 dozen.

PEANUT BUTTER COOKIES

- **½ cup corn-free margarine**
- **½ cup corn-free brown sugar**
- **½ cup corn-free white sugar**
- **½ teaspoon vanilla**
- **½ teaspoon salt**
- **1 teaspoon baking soda**
- **1½ cups El Molino soya carob flour**
- **½ cup peanut butter**
- **1 EGG**

Cream margarine, sugars, vanilla, salt and baking soda. Add peanut butter and egg. Mix dry ingredients together and work in. Shape into balls, place on greased cookie sheet and press down or flatten with prongs of fork. Bake at 375°F. from 10 to 12 minutes. Makes about 2 dozen.

Meringue

MACAROON MERINGUE

- **1 tablespoon CORN-STARCH**
- **6 EGG whites**
- **1 cup sugar**
- **¼ pound blanched almonds**
- **1 cup sherry**
- **24 macaroons**

Add cornstarch to egg yolks and beat well. Add sugar and almonds. Add sherry. Heat in double boiler, stirring constantly until thickened. Arrange macaroons on shallow baking dish. Cover with sauce. Spread meringue on top and brown in oven at 250°F. for approximately 50 minutes. Makes approximately 3 cups.

Pie

LEMON PIE

- 6 teaspoons Jolly Joan Egg Replacer
- 6 tablespoons warm water
- 1 cup sugar
- ¼ cup CORNSTARCH
- ⅛ teaspoon salt
- 1¼ cups hot water
- 2 teaspoons grated lemon rind
- ¼ cup lemon juice
- 1 tablespoon vegetable oil
- 1 baked 9-inch pie shell

Place egg replacer in a mixing bowl ard slowly add warm water. Beat until fluffy. In a double boiler combine sugar, cornstarch and salt. Gradually pour in hot water, lemon rind and juice. Cook, stirring, over high heat. Add 3 tablespoons of mixture from double boiler to egg replacer and beat until fluffy. Pour back into double boiler, stirring thoroughly. Add vegetable oil and continue stirring over high heat until smooth and thick enough to mound when dropped from spoon. Cool 5 minutes, then pour into pie shell. Cool thoroughly and serve plain or topped with soy whipped cream. Serves 8 to 10.

Puddings

GRAPE JUICE SPONGE

- ½ cup cold water
- 1 envelope gelatin
- ⅓ cup sugar
- ¼ teaspoon salt
- 1 cup grape juice, heated
- 1 tablespoon lemon juice
- 2 EGG whites, stiffly beaten

Pour cold water in bowl and sprinkle gelatin on top. Add sugar, salt and hot grape juice, stirring until dissolved. Add lemon juice and cool. When jelly begins to thicken, beat until frothy. Fold in egg whites. Turn into mold that has been rinsed in cold water and chill. When firm, unmold. Garnish with bits of fruit. Makes approximately 2 cups.

HAMBURG CREAM

5 EGGS, separated
Juice and grated rind of 2 lemons
1 cup sugar, sifted

Beat egg yolks until thick. Add lemon juice and rind, then sugar. Cook in double boiler until stiff. Beat egg whites until stiff and fold in. Chill in sherbet glasses before serving. Serves 6.

PEACH SNOWBALLS

¼ cup cold water
1 envelope gelatin
¼ cup sugar
¼ teaspoon salt
½ cup hot water or hot canned peach juice
2 tablespoons lemon juice
1 cup canned peaches (or apricots or pineapple)
2 EGG whites, stiffly beaten

Pour gelatin over cold water in a bowl. Add sugar, salt and hot water. Stir until gelatin and sugar are dissolved. Add lemon juice and peaches pressed through a sieve. Cool. When mixture begins to thicken, beat until frothy, then fold in egg whites. Turn into small molds which have been rinsed in cold water. Chill.

PRUNE WHIP

¼ cup cold water
1 envelope gelatin
½ cup sugar
¼ teaspoon salt
¾ cup prune juice, heated
2 tablespoons lemon juice
1 cup prune pulp
2 EGG whites, stiffly beaten

Pour cold water in bowl and sprinkle gelatin on top. Add sugar, salt and prune juice, stirring until gelatin is dissolved. Add lemon juice and prune pulp. Cool. When mixture begins to thicken fold in egg whites. Turn into sherbet glasses or into mold that has been rinsed in cold water. Serves 4 to 6.

SAUCES AND GRAVIES

MEDIUM CREAM SAUCE WITH RICE FLOUR
(See recipe Part 13)

RYE FLOUR GRAVY (See recipe Part 13)

HORSERADISH SAUCE

¼ onion, finely chopped (optional)
2 tablespoons chicken fat
2 tablespoons CORNSTARCH
3 tablespoons grated horseradish
1 cup soup stock, heated (or water)
2 tablespoons vinegar
2 cloves (optional)
2 bay leaves
½ teaspoon salt
⅛ teaspoon pepper (optional)
2 tablespoons sugar

Fry onion in fat until brown. Blend in cornstarch and horseradish. Gradually add the soup stock and when smooth, the remaining ingredients. Cook 5 minutes more, remove bay leaves, and, if desired, add more horseradish, sugar or vinegar. Makes approximately 1¾ cups.

SAUCE FOR FISH

1 tablespoon olive oil
1 tablespoon CORNSTARCH
2 cups stewed tomatoes
1 teaspoon vinegar
½ teaspoon sugar
Salt
Sliced green pepper

Mix ingredients in order. Boil until thickened, stirring to prevent lumps. Makes approximately 2 cups.

TOMATO SAUCE

1 onion, chopped
1 tablespoon olive oil
1 tablespoon CORN-STARCH
1 cup tomato puree
½ teaspoon sugar
1 teaspoon vinegar
Salt and pepper
1 teaspoon catsup

In a frying pan brown onion in oil. Add cornstarch, which has been thinned in water, to tomato puree. Add sugar, vinegar, salt and pepper, then catsup. Thicken. Serve hot. Makes approximately 1¼ cups.

SECTION IV

WHEAT ALLERGY

INTRODUCTION

When interest in food allergies entered the phase of science rather than conjecture, wheat, eggs and milk were found to be far and away the leading offenders among the vast array of edible ingestants. The fact that corn has probably passed wheat in the last two or three decades does not diminish the importance of wheat as much as it adds a new allergen.

Many thousands of varieties of wheat have been grown in the world. Sensitivity to one means sensitivity to all. Wheat is so often a contaminant of other flours that one who is very sensitive to wheat has to be careful. In one study rye flours were found to be as much as 5% wheat flour.

People highly allergic to wheat may develop allergies to other grains more easily than to, say, watermelon. It is always best to alternate other grains in the diet from week to week, if they have proven to be non-allergic at first.

Wheat may cause trouble as an ingestant, an inhalant or by contact. When it bothers people only by inhalation, hypoimmunization, may be successful. Less often a skin rash from contact will submit to the same treatment. Otherwise avoidance of wheat is necessary. Foods prepared in the home or elsewhere can be contaminated with wheat in the cooking process. Stuffing in a turkey contaminates the meat. A spoon dropped in a flour gravy should not be used to stir something else. In a restaurant ask for "pure" foods—no gravy, no sauce.

Of the remaining widely used cereal grains rice is the least antigenic, especially if polished and not made shiny with corn syrup. In ascending order of severity are wild rice, oats, barley and rye.

The following list contains many of the possible contact with wheat. Remember there are others!

Wheat is found in the following foods:

Beverages:
- Beer*
- Cocomalt
- Gin (any drink containing grain neutral spirits)
- Malted milk
- Ovaltine
- Postum
- Whiskies

Breads:
- Biscuits
- Cornbread**
- Crackers
- Gluten bread
- Graham bread
- Muffins
- Popovers
- Pretzels
- Pumpernickel bread
- Rolls
- Rye bread
- Soy bread
- White bread
- (see Note No. 1)

Cereals:
- Bran flakes
- Cornflakes
- Crackels
- Cream of Wheat
- Farina
- Grapenuts
- Krumbles
- Muffets
- Pep
- Pettijohn's
- Puffed wheat
- Ralston's Wheat Cereal
- Rice Krispies
- Shredded Wheat
- Triscuits
- Wheatena and many other malted cereals

Flours:
- Buckwheat flour**
- Corn flour**
- Gluten flour
- Graham flour
- Flour
- Lima bean flour*
- Paten flour
- Rice flour**
- Rye flour
- White flour
- Whole-wheat flour
- One should not overlook mixtures with flour in them!

Miscellaneous:
- Bologna
- Bouillon cubes
- Chocolate candy
- Chocolate except, bitter cocoa and chocolate
- Cooked mixed meat dishes
- Fats used for frying foods rolled in flour
- Fish rolled in flour
- Fowl rolled in flour
- Gravies
- Griddle cakes
- Hamburger, etc.
- Hotcakes
- Ice cream cones

*There are some kinds free of wheat.
**Unless homemade without wheat.

- Liverwurst
- Lunch ham
- Malt products or foods containing malt
- Matzos
- Mayonnaise**
- Meat rolled in flour (do not overlook meat fried in frying fat which has been used to fry meats rolled in flour—particularly in restaurants!)
- Most cooked sausages
- Pancake mixtures
- Sauces
- Some yeasts
- Synthetic pepper
- Thickening in ice creams
- Waffles
- Wheat cakes
- Wheat germ
- Wieners

Pastries and Desserts:

- Cakes
- Candy bars
- Chocolate candy
- Cookies**
- Doughnuts
- Frozen pies
- Pies
- Puddings

Wheat Products:

- Bread and cracker crumbs
- Dumplings
- Hamburger mix
- Macaroni
- Noodles
- Rusk
- Spaghetti
- Vermicelli
- Zwieback

Important: Prepare foods in separate containers without contact-stuffings, dressings, sauces, gravies, steam cooking and frying fats! Study the labels of all foods and determine if they contain wheat. Do not expect the menu in restaurants to be accurate—anticipate this when ordering.

Do not use: Rye, wheatless mixes, "Accent," "Zest," or monosodium glutamate UNLESS specifically instructed to do so.

Note No. 1: Rye products are not entirely free of wheat. Whether you can use rye will have to be studied as an individual problem, if you are found sensitive to wheat.

Note No. 2: The inclusion of malted cereals in the wheat list is due to the fact that for purposes of clinical procedure, barley is considered as being identical with wheat. There, however, definite sensitizations to barley malt when allergy to wheat cannot be proven. The reverse is also occasionally true!

**Some preparations can be obtained free of wheat.

PART 15

No Wheat

APPETIZERS

SARDINE FINGERS

4 sardines, chopped
½ cup soy BUTTER
Horseradish
Rye potato bread*
Sliced, stuffed olives

Cream together sardines and butter. Add horseradish to taste. Cut bread into finger lengths and spread with paste. Arrange olives in an overlapping row down the center. Makes about ¾ cup.

*See recipe under Breads, Part 9.

SARDINE SANDWICH

1 (3.75-ounce) can sardines
Juice of 1 lemon
Salt and pepper
2 tablespoons soy BUTTER, melted
Rye Potato Bread*

Chop sardines to fine paste. Add lemon juice, seasonings, and butter. Spread between thin slices of buttered Rye Potato Bread. Makes about ¾ cup.

*See recipe under Breads, Part 9.

BLACK-EYED SUSAN

4 EGG hard-cooked yolks
½ cup BUTTER, softened
4 drops Tabasco
¼ teaspoon salt
⅛ teaspoon pepper
¼ teaspoon onion juice
16 rye wafers
1 (3-ounce) can caviar

Press egg yolks through a sieve. Add butter, Tabasco, salt, pepper and onion juice, blending together until smooth. Spread on rye wafers. Put a dab of caviar in center of each. Makes 16.

CHICKEN LIVERS SAUTÉED

Chicken livers
BUTTER or chicken fat
Salt
Rye wafers

Wash chicken livers and slice, allowing one or more to each rye wafer. Brown livers in butter. Season with salt. Serve on hot buttered rye wafers. Prepare desired number.

ANCHOVY PASTE ON POTATO CHIPS (See recipe Part 1)

MUSHROOM CANAPÉS

10 mushrooms, finely chopped
BUTTER
½ cup heavy CREAM
¼ teaspoon CORNSTARCH
Seasonings
Rye Melba toast

Sauté mushrooms in butter for 5 minutes. Heat with cream, to which has been added the cornstarch thinned with a little cream. Season to taste. Spread on rye Melba toast. Makes about ¾ cup.

OLIVES

Pimola **½ slice bacon**

Wrap a large pimola in ½ slice hot crisp bacon. Fasten with toothpick. Makes 1.

CREAM CHEESE CANAPÉ

CREAM CHEESE
Mayonnaise
Rye wafers
Chopped pecans

Season cream cheese with homemade mayonnaise. Spread on rye wafers. Sprinkle with pecans. Prepare desired amount.

BREADS

RYE BREAD (See recipe Part 4)

ORANGE SOYBEAN BREAD (See recipe Part 4)

RYE MUFFINS (See recipe Part 4)

SOY BEAN MUFFINS (See recipe Part 4)

SOY BEAN PANCAKES (See recipe Part 4)

RICE WAFFLES (See recipe Part 4)

WAFFLES (See recipe Part 4)

RYE BAKING POWDER BREAD (See recipe Part 11)

EGGLESS NUT BREAD (See recipe Part 11)

BARLEY BREAD (See recipe Part 11)

CORNBREAD (See recipe Part 11)

RYE AND CORN MEAL MUFFINS (See recipe Part 11)

CORNMEAL CAKES (See recipe Part 11)

PANCAKES (See recipe Part 11)

RICE AND RYE FLOUR BREAD (See recipe Part 12)

RYE BREAD (See recipe Part 12)

SOUTHERN CONE PONE (See recipe Part 12)

CROUTONS (See recipe Part 12)

CINNAMON TOAST (See recipe Part 12)

RICE MUFFINS (See recipe Part 12)

SOYALAC PANCAKES (See recipe Part 12)

SOYALAC CORN STICKS (See recipe Part 12)

BISCUITS APPLE STYLE (See recipe Part 1)

BARLEY RYE BREAD

1½ cups whole barley flour
⅓ cup whole rye FLOUR
⅛ teaspoon salt
1 tablespoon baking powder
¼ cup MILK
2 teaspoons BUTTER
1 tablespoon honey
2 EGG whites, beaten

Sift flour before measuring. Mix dry ingredients. Combine milk, butter and honey and add to dry ingredients. Beat well. Fold in egg whites. Bake in a 4x5x2-inch pan in a 350°F. oven for 15 minutes. Makes 1 loaf.

OAT BREAD

1⅓ cups whole oat flour
¼ teaspoon salt
1 tablespoon baking powder
2 teaspoons corn-free margarine
⅓ cup water
1 EGG

Sift flour before measuring. Mix dry ingredients, and cut in margarine. Beat egg and water, mix with dry ingredients and beat well. Bake in a 4x7x2-inch pan at 375°F. for 30 minutes. Makes 1 loaf.

QUICK-RAISED RICE BREAD

2 EGGS*
1 cup soy milk
2 tablespoons vegetable oil
2 tablespoons sugar
2 cups Jolly Joan Rice Mix

Separate eggs and beat whites until stiff. In a separate bowl beat yolks, then add milk, oil and sugar. Add rice mix and stir until smooth. Gently fold in egg whites until batter is mixed. Pour in 8x4x2-inch bread pan and place in center of a preheated 350°F. oven. Bake for 45 minutes, or until brown. Turn out on wire rack until cool. Makes 1 loaf.

*Or use Jolly Joan Egg Replacer

CORN BREAD

¾ cup CORNMEAL
¾ cup scalded MILK
⅓ teaspoon salt
1 tablespoon BUTTER, melted
1 EGG, beaten

Mix ingredients. Pour into a greased dish. Bake at 400°F. for 20 minutes, or until brown. Makes about 1¾ cups.

HOMINY GRITS BREAD

- 2 cups cold hominy grits
- 1 cup CORNMEAL
- 2 cups MILK
- 2 EGGS, separated
- 1 teaspoon salt
- 1 teaspoon baking powder
- 2 teaspoons BUTTER

Mash grits until free from lumps. Scald meal with hot milk and mix thoroughly with grits. Add egg yolks and salt. Stiffly beat egg whites and fold in. Stir baking powder in last. Dot top with butter. Bake in a preheated 300°F. oven for 25 to 35 minutes, or until consistency of custard is reached. Makes about 5½ cups.

SONORA STYLE CORN BREAD

- 1 cup CORNMEAL
- ½ teaspoon baking soda
- 1 teaspoon salt
- 2 EGGS
- 1 cup MILK
- 1 (1 pound) can cream-style CORN
- 5 strips bacon, cut in 2-inch pieces
- ¼ pound American CHEESE, grated
- 1 small onion, diced
- 1 (7-ounce) can diced chili peppers

Blend cornmeal, soda, salt in a mixing bowl. Beat eggs and milk together. Add corn to cornmeal, then add milk and eggs. Fry bacon and add drippings only to batter. Pour half the batter into a greased 8x8x2-inch square baking dish. Combine cheese, onion and peppers and scatter over batter. Pour in rest of batter and top with bacon. Bake in a preheated 350°F. oven for 45 to 60 minutes. Serve hot. Serves 8.

VIRGINIA SPOON BREAD

- **2 cups CORNMEAL, scalded**
- **1 quart BUTTERMILK**
- **1 teaspoon baking soda**
- **2 tablespoons BUTTER**
- **4 EGGS, beaten**
- **½ teaspoon baking powder**
- **¾ teaspoon salt**

Thin the cornmeal with buttermilk, in which soda has been dissolved, to consistency of a batter for cakes. Melt butter in pan in which bread is to be baked. Add, with eggs, baking powder and salt, to mixture. After stirring well pour into hot pan and bake quickly in a 450°F. oven for 50 to 55 minutes. When well browned, serve hot from pan with spoon. Makes about 1¾ quarts.

RYE ROLLS

- **¼ cup sugar**
- **2 tablespoons BUTTER**
- **¼ teaspoon salt**
- **¼ cup boiling water**
- **1 EGG**
- **¼ cup cold water**
- **½ cake compressed wheat-free yeast**
- **2 tablespoons lukewarm water**
- **1½ cups rye FLOUR**
- **½ cup CORNSTARCH**

Melt sugar, butter and salt with boiling water. Mix egg and cold water. Add to mixture yeast dissolved in lukewarm water. Sift together rye flour and cornstarch, after measuring, then stir in. Refrigerate for at least 8 hours. Remove and shape dough. Allow to rise for 4 hours at 80°F. Bake in a preheated oven 450°F. for 30 minutes. Makes about 2 dozen.

BISCUITS

2 tablespoons CORNMEAL
½ cup rye FLOUR
¾ teaspoon baking powder
1/16 teaspoon salt
1 teaspoon BUTTER
2 tablespoons MILK (more if needed)

Sift together dry ingredients, then add remaining ingredients. Form into balls the size of a walnut. Drop on a buttered cookie sheet and press flat. Bake in a 450°F. oven for 25 minutes. Makes 7 small biscuits.

OAT BISCUITS

½ tablespoon shortening
½ cup Scotch oats (ground oatmeal)
1 tablespoon CORNSTARCH
1 teaspoon baking powder
⅛ teaspoon salt
1 tablespoon MILK (or more)

Mix shortening with dry ingredients, then add milk to make soft dough. Pat into round biscuits. Bake in a preheated 350°F. oven for 35 minutes. Makes 6 small biscuits.

MUFFINS

¼ cup CORNSTARCH
½ cup soybean FLOUR
1 teaspoon salt
2 teaspoons baking powder
4 EGGS, separated

Sift dry ingredients together. Add 1 to 2 tablespoons water to moisten egg yolks. Beat. Beat egg whites until stiff and fold in. Half fill greased muffin tins. Bake in a preheated 400°F. oven for about 20 to 30 minutes. Makes 8 to 10.

WAFFLES

- **1 EGG**
- **½ cup MILK**
- **1 tablespoon BUTTER, melted**
- **½ cup CORNMEAL**
- **2 tablespoons CORNSTARCH**
- **1 teaspoon sugar**
- **½ cup potato flour**
- **1 teaspoon baking powder**
- **pinch of salt**

Combine ingredients. Preheat electric iron for 10 minutes. Allow 4 minutes for cooking each waffle. Makes 2.

APPLE WAFFLES

- **⅔ cup soybean FLOUR**
- **⅓ cup CORNSTARCH**
- **½ teaspoon sugar**
- **⅓ teaspoon cinnamon**
- **1½ teaspoons baking powder**
- **¾ cup MILK**
- **1 EGG, separated**
- **1 cup finely grated apples**
- **2 tablespoons BUTTER, melted**

Sift together dry ingredients, then add milk and beaten egg yolk. When smooth, add apples and pour in butter. Beat egg white until stiff and fold in. Preheat electric iron for 10 minutes. Allow 4 minutes for cooking each waffle. Makes 2 or 3.

SOYBEAN WAFFLES

- **⅓ cup soybean FLOUR**
- **1 tablespoon CORNSTARCH**
- **¾ teaspoon baking powder**
- **⅛ teaspoon salt**
- **½ cup MILK (or water)**
- **1 EGG, beaten**
- **1 teaspoon shortening, melted**

Sift dry ingredients, then add remaining ingredients in order. Preheat electric iron for 10 minutes. Allow 4 minutes for cooking each waffle. Makes 1.

RICE-POTATO WAFFLE

1½ cups rice FLOUR
2 cups potato starch
2 teaspoons salt
2 teaspoons baking powder
2½ cups MILK
4 EGGS, separated
6 tablespoons BUTTER, melted

Sift dry ingredients. Add milk and beaten egg yolks, then butter. Beat egg whites until stiff and fold in. Bake in a hot waffle iron. Makes 4 to 6.

WAFFLES WITH RICE FLOUR

3½ cups rice FLOUR
2 teaspoons baking powder
2 teaspoons salt
3 cups MILK
4 EGGS, separated
6 tablespoons BUTTER, melted

Sift dry ingredients together. Add milk, beaten egg yolks and butter. Beat egg whites until stiff and fold in. Bake in a hot waffle iron. Serve with melted butter and syrup. Makes 4 to 6.

FRENCH PANCAKES

½ cup CORNSTARCH
1½ cups soybean FLOUR
1¼ cups MILK
2 EGGS, well beaten
Wine or vanilla to taste
½ tablespoon olive oil
¼ teaspoon salt

Sift together cornstarch and flour. Mix in a little milk and add the eggs. Flavor with wine, then add oil and salt. Beat well. Add remainder of milk, beating with a spoon. Let the batter stand in a cool place for 2 hours. Cook on a greased griddle. Serve immediately on hot plates. Dust with confectioners' sugar, or cover half cake with jam and fold over like a small omelet. Makes 1 dozen, depending on size.

BATTER DIP, WITH EGG REPLACER

6 teaspoons Jolly Joan Egg Replacer
6 tablespoons warm water
Rye or potato FLOUR or crumbs

Add replacer slowly to warm water. Mix thoroughly and beat until fluffy. Dip pieces of chicken, etc., in this mixture until thoroughly coated. Then dip in flour or crumbs. Mixture may be brushed on with pastry brush if you prefer. Pan fry or deep fry in your favorite manner.

CEREALS

CORNMEAL MUSH (See recipe Part 12)

GRITS (See recipe Part 12)

OATMEAL (See recipe Part 12)

HOMINY GRITS

1 cup hominy grits
1 teaspoon salt
6 cups boiling water

Cook in a double boiler for at least 1 hour. Stir from time to time to avoid lumps forming. Serves 4 to 6.

OATMEAL

2 cups water
Salt to taste
Instant oat flakes
Sherry or port

Bring water to a brisk boil in a pan over direct heat. Salt to taste. Stir in 1 cup instant oat flakes and boil slowly for 3 minutes. To alter thickness of mixture add more or less water. Serves 4.

Note: Sherry or port wine added to oatmeal gruel gives a delicious flavor and imparts additional food value.

RICE RING

1 cup uncooked rice
1½ quarts boiling water
1 teaspoon salt
1 EGG, beaten
1 tablespoon BUTTER, melted
1 tablespoon Worcestershire sauce
2 tablespoon CREAM
⅛ teaspoon pepper (optional)

Cover rice with boiling water. Add salt and simmer until tender but not mushy, about 25 minutes. Drain and rinse with cold water. Drain again. Add egg, butter, Worcestershire sauce, cream, salt and pepper. Place in greased ring mold and set in pan one-fourth full of warm water. Bake in a 350°F. oven until mixture is firm, about 45 minutes. Unmold on round platter. Serves 4 or 5.

SOUPS

PEA SOUP

- **2 cups cooked peas**
- **1 cup liquid, from peas**
- **2 slices onion**
- **1 stalk celery, chopped**
- **1 small carrot**
- **3/16 teaspoon pepper (optional)**
- **3 tablespoons BUTTER**
- **3 tablespoons CORN-STARCH**
- **½ teaspoon salt**
- **1¾ cups evaporated MILK**
- **2¼ cups water**

Cook first five ingredients until soft. Add ⅛ teaspoon pepper. Blend with butter, cornstarch, salt, remaining pepper, evaporated milk and water. Combine cornstarch, butter and milk to make sauce. Reheat with vegetables. Makes about 1¾ quarts.

CREAM OF MUSHROOM SOUP

- **½ pound mushrooms**
- **1 quart chicken or veal broth**
- **1 slice onion (or garlic salt)**
- **2 tablespoons BUTTER**
- **2 tablespoons rice FLOUR**
- **1 cup CREAM**
- **Salt and pepper (optional)**

Chop mushrooms very fine. Add to broth with onion and cook for 20 minutes. Rub through a sieve and reheat. Melt butter in saucepan and add flour. When it bubbles add ⅔ cup mushrooms and soup liquid. Stir in the rest, then add the cream and seasonings. Makes about 1½ cups.

CREAM OF OYSTER SOUP

2 cups oyster liquor
1 cup MILK
1 cup CREAM
Salt and pepper
2 tablespoons BUTTER
Parsley
12 to 16 oysters
1 tablespoon potato flour

Put oyster liquor on stove in a saucepan and combine milk and cream in a double boiler. When liquor boils, skim. Season with salt, pepper, butter and parsley. Just before serving drop oysters in liquor. Boil just long enough to get plump. Thicken the cream with potato flour that has been moistened with a little milk. Makes about 1 quart.

BARLEY SOUP

½ cup pearl barley
1 quart boiling water
1 teaspoon salt
2 quarts soup stock
⅛ teaspoon pepper (optional)

Wash barley in cold water. Cook in boiling salted water until tender, ½ hour or more. When water has evaporated, add soup stock. Cook 45 minutes longer. Season.

GUMBO

1 quart tomatoes
2 cups okra
1 large onion (optional)
2 green peppers
½ cup bacon fat
Salt
Pepper (optional)

Peel and cup up tomatoes, okra, onion and peppers. Fry in bacon fat until brown. Season with salt and pepper. Cook slowly, for approximately 50 to 60 minutes, adding no water. Serve with rice.

CHICKEN SOUP WITH RICE

1 (3- to 4-pound) chicken
3 to 4 quarts water
1 tablespoon salt
1 onion
2 stalks celery
¼ cup diced celery root
¼ teaspoon pepper
2 tablespoons cooked rice

Select an old hen. Singe, clean and cut up. Salt and let stand for several hours. Cover with cold water and bring to a boil quickly. Skim thoroughly. Simmer 3 hours or more. Add the vegetables and simmer 1 hour longer. Strain, remove fat (save for frying) and season to taste. Add rice before serving. When chicken is tender, use for salads, croquettes or serve with arrowroot sauce.* Serves 6 to 8.

*See following recipe

ARROWROOT SAUCE

1 tablespoon arrowroot powder
2 tablespoons BUTTER
¾ cup MILK

Blend arrowroot and butter together to a smooth paste. Add milk a little at a time until sauce is correct consistency.

BALLS FOR SOUP

3 heaping tablespoons Swedish rye or rye cracker crumbs
1 heaping tablespoon chicken fat
1 EGG
2 tablespoons ice water
Chopped parsley
Seasonings

Roll to crumbs 1 slice Swedish rye or 6 rye crackers. Combine 3 heaping tablespoons crumbs, chicken fat, egg, ice water, parsley and seasonings. Place in refrigerator for 4 hours. Take ¾ teaspoon of this mixture and roll in palm of hand. Continue until all mixture is used. Boil, uncovered, for 30 minutes.

CREAMED FRESH PEA SOUP (See recipe Part 13)

TOMATO CREAM SOUP (See recipe Part 13)

MULL-SOY VEGETABLE CREAM SOUP (See recipe Part 13)

TOMATO SOUP (See recipe Part 13)

CHICKEN SOUP

1 (3- to 4-pound) fowl
1 tablespoon salt
3 to 4 quarts water
1 onion (optional)
2 stalks celery
¼ cup diced celery root
¼ teaspoon pepper (optional)
CORNSTARCH sauce (optional)

Select an old hen. Singe, clean and cut up. Salt and let stand for several hours. Cover with cold water and bring to a boil quickly. Skim thoroughly. Simmer 3 hours or more. Add vegetables, and simmer 1 hour longer. Strain, remove fat (save for frying) and season to taste. When chicken is tender, cut up for salads, croquettes or serve with arrowroot sauce. Serves 4 to 6.

Note: See notes in Part 9 introduction and Miscellaneous Part 16.

FISH

CRABS À LA CREOLE

6 crabs
1 small onion, chopped
1 tablespoon chicken fat
1 tablespoon CORNSTARCH
1 cup hot water
2 cups tomato puree
Salt and pepper (optional)
½ teaspoon sugar
1 tablespoon catsup

Cook live crabs in boiling water until red. Remove from heat, pick out meat carefully from claws and body and set aside. In a saucepan, brown onion in chicken fat. Stir in cornstarch, hot water and tomato puree. Season with salt and pepper, sugar and catsup. Boil until thick. Add crabmeat and let cook a few minutes. Serves 3 to 4.

GUMBO À LA CREOLE

Garlic, chopped, or large onion
Soy BUTTER or fat
1 quart sliced okra
1 pound lake shrimps, boiled and cleaned
2 quarts hot water
1 pound beef brisket (optional)
CORNMEAL
1 pound canned tomatoes
6 crabs, boiled and cleaned
Salt, pepper and bay leaf
6 to 8 tablespoons cooked rice

Brown garlic or onion in butter. Add okra and cook until browned. Add shrimp and brown again. Put into a soup pot and cover with hot water. Season brisket, dredge with cornmeal and brown on both sides in fat. Add to the soup. Add tomato and crabs (the claws and bodies should be broken). Add seasoning last. Cover pot and allow to simmer for 2 hours. When ready to serve, remove bay leaf and place some of the crab in each soup plate with serving of gumbo. A tablespoon of rice is served with each helping. Serves 6 to 8.

BAKED TROUT

1 tablespoon CORNSTARCH
1 cup stewed tomatoes
Juice from tomatoes
3½ pounds trout
Salt and pepper
1 onion, chopped
1 stalk celery, chopped
1 tablespoon BUTTER
Worcestershire sauce

Wet cornstarch with several tablespoons of tomato juice. Season fish. Combine fish with all ingredients except cornstarch.

Bake in a preheated 375°F. oven for 30 minutes, basting occasionally. When done thicken sauce with cornstarch and pour over fish. Serve hot. Serves 4.

BUTTERFISH SAUTÉ

Fish
Salt and pepper
CORNFLAKES or CORNMEAL
Fat

Clean fish and season with salt and pepper. Dip in crushed cornflakes or cornmeal. Heat fat and fry fish golden brown. Turn and brown other side. (Sautéing requires less fat than frying.) Prepare portions desired.

COQUILLE OF FISH

1 pound fish (any kind)
2 tablespoons BUTTER, melted
1 tablespoon CORNSTARCH
Pinch of cayenne
1 cup MILK
1 tablespoon anchovy paste or Worcestershire sauce
Pinch of salt
CORNFLAKE crumbs

Boil and shred fish. Melt butter in a saucepan and stir in cornstarch and cayenne. Stir in milk, anchovy paste and salt. Let thicken, stirring constantly. Remove from heat and stir in fish. Line greased individual shells or one large greased pudding dish with fried cornflake crumbs. Fill with mixture and sprinkle fried cornflake crumbs on top. Bake in hot oven until brown. Serves 2 to 3.

Note: Salmon can also be used.

SCALLOPED FISH

- **2 tablespoons fat**
- **1 cup crushed CORNFLAKES**
- **2 pounds fish, cut into 2½-inch cubes**
- **Tomato sauce, heated**
- **Parsley**
- **Lemon slices**
- **¼ cup finely chopped almonds**

Melt fat and combine with cornflakes. Put fish cubes in greased baking dish. Cover with hot tomato sauce and sprinkle cornflakes on top. Bake in a preheated 450°F. oven for 15 to 20 minutes, or until flakes are browned. Decorate with parsley, lemon slices and almonds. Serves 4 or 5.

LOBSTER DELMONICO

- **1 (2-pound) lobster**
- **½ teaspoon salt**
- **¼ cup BUTTER**
- **1 cup CREAM**
- **2 level teaspoons CORNSTARCH**
- **Cayenne (optional)**
- **2 EGG yolks**
- **2 tablespoons sherry**

Boil lobster in salted water for 20 minutes. Cut meat in small cubes. Keep lobster hot in a double boiler. Melt butter and add cream. Thicken with cornstarch, which has been thinned with a little cool water. Season with cayenne. Cook, stirring constantly, until mixture is smooth, about 2 minutes. Add egg yolks to cream mixture, then add sherry. Pour over lobster. Serve hot. Serves 4.

MEAT

MEATBALLS

2 cups tomato sauce
Pinch of salt and pepper
Pinch of garlic
Pinch of basil or oregano
Parsley sprigs
2 pounds ground meat
2 slices stale rye bread
2 EGGS
¼ cup rice FLOUR
Olive oil

Make a sauce of first five ingredients. Combine meat, bread, and eggs (this should be sticky). Make balls of meat and roll lightly in rice flour. Brown in a little olive oil. Add to sauce. Simmer on top of stove at very low heat all day, stirring frequently so it does not stick to bottom of pan. Serves 6.

MEAT-RICE PATTIES

½ pound ground beef
½ to ¾ teaspoon salt
¾ cup cooked rice
¼ cup Mull-Soy

Combine all ingredients. Shape into patties, using ¼ cup mixture for each patty. Place on broiler pan, 3 inches from heat, and cook until browned. Turn and brown on other side. Serve hot. Makes 6 patties.

SWISS STEAK

1 teaspoon salt
½ teaspoon pepper
½ cup potato flour
2½ pounds round steak
2 tablespoons chicken fat
½ onion, chopped
½ green pepper, seeded and finely chopped
1½ cups water
½ cup catsup

Add salt and pepper to flour. Pound into meat. Brown in skillet with fat. Add onion, green pepper, water and catsup. Cover tightly and simmer slowly until tender, about 2 hours. You may also cook in oven, at 350°F. for 1 hour if desired. Serves 4 to 6.

HAM POTATO CASSEROLE

4 medium-sized potatoes
2 cups diced baked ham
2 tablespoons chopped green pepper
Pepper
Dash of garlic salt
2 tablespoons soy margarine
2 tablespoons rice FLOUR
1¼ cups Sobee liquid
1¼ cups water

Arrange peeled and thinly sliced potatoes in alternate layers with ham in baking dish, which has been greased with corn-free fat. Add green pepper, pepper and garlic salt. Make a white sauce of the last four ingredients and pour over potatoes and ham so the sauce reaches the bottom of the dish. Place on center rack of oven. Bake in a 400°F. oven for about 1 hour, or until potatoes are tender when pierced with a fork. Serves 4.

MEAT LOAF (See recipe Part 9)

HAMBURGER PATTIE (See recipe Part 9)

POULTRY

CHICKEN BAKED WITH OYSTERS (See recipe Part 13)

MEXICANA CHICKEN (See recipe Part 13)

FRIED CHICKEN

1 (3-to 3½-pound) chicken
Potato flour
Salt and pepper
Corn-free oil

Wash, dry and disjoint chicken. Dredge in flour seasoned with salt and pepper. Fry in oil about ¾ to 1-inch deep. Turn constantly to brown. Cover and cook slowly for about 45 minutes. Serves 4.

CAPON

1 (4 to 5-pound) capon
Hoecake Stuffing*

Prepare capon as usual. Stuff with hoecake stuffing. Serves 4 to 6.

*See following recipe.

POULTRY STUFFING

*HOECAKE STUFFING

Hoecake
Celery
Gizzard (and liver) of fowl
Soup stock
CORNMEAL
1 EGG
Salt and pepper

Make Hoecake. Crumble. Cut celery. Stew in water with gizzard until tender. Chop gizzard (and liver, if desired). Add to soup stock, or liquid from celery. Mix with cornmeal to desired consistency, add egg and seasoning. Stuff and bake chicken.

*See recipe under Poultry Stuffing, Part 9.

APPLE STUFFING

1 teaspoon paprika
¼ teaspoon pepper
¼ teaspoon cinnamon
⅛ teaspoon cloves
1½ teaspoons salt
½ teaspoon celery salt
4 cups Swedish rye crumbs
½ cup BUTTER
1 cup boiling water
4 cups chopped apples
1 cup chopped celery
1 medium-sized onion, chopped

Mix seasonings and crumbs. Add butter to water with remaining ingredients, blending thoroughly. Makes about 10 cups.

Note: Any or all spices may be omitted.

VEGETABLES

BOILED ONIONS

Onions (use desired quantity)
White Sauce (recipe follows)
Salted water

Peel onions under cold water. Put in saucepan with boiling salted water (1 teaspoon salt to 1 quart water). Boil for 5 minutes, drain. Again cover with boiling water. Cook 1 hour, or until soft. Drain. Cover with white sauce.

WHITE SAUCE

1 tablespoon potato flour
1 tablespoon BUTTER
1 cup MILK (or corn-free vegetable liquor)
Salt and pepper

Blend flour and butter. Add liquid, stirring until smooth. Makes about 1 cup.

SARATOGA ONIONS

Onions (use desired quantity)
MILK
Rice FLOUR
Fat

Slice onions crosswise into rings. Separate each ring. Dip in milk. Drain, then dredge with flour and fry in deep hot fat a few at a time until brown and crisp. Serve as a border with roast or steak.

SCALLOPED POTATOES

2 cups raw potatoes (about 6 to 8)
1 teaspoon salt
¼ teaspoon pepper (optional)
4 tablespoons BUTTER
3 tablespoons rice FLOUR
2 cups scalded MILK

Cover the bottom of a buttered baking dish with a layer of sliced potatoes, sprinkle with salt and pepper, dot with pieces of butter and dredge with flour. Repeat until the ingredients are used. Pour scalded milk over all. Bake in a 350°F. oven for 45 to 50 minutes. Serves 4 to 6.

EGGPLANT

1 eggplant
Rice or potato FLOUR
Salt
Soy BUTTER or safflower margarine
1 onion, sliced thin
Salt and pepper to taste
Pinch of marjoram

Cut eggplant into thin slices. Soak in salted water to cover, weighted down with a plate (eggplant will rise to surface if not weighted). Remove, wash and dry slices. Dredge in mixture of flour and salt. Melt shortening and coat eggplant slices on both sides with it. Then add the onion and seasonings. Bake in a 400°F. oven for about 15 minutes or until tender. Turn once when bottom is brown. Serve very hot. Serves 4.

BAKED TOMATOES

1½ teaspoons salt
1½ teaspoons sugar
1½ teaspoons grated onion (optional)
3½ cups cooked (or canned) tomatoes
2¾ cups CORNFLAKES
5 tablespoons BUTTER

Add salt, sugar and onion (omit onion, if allergic) to tomatoes. Alternate layers of cornflakes, butter and tomatoes in a greased baking dish. Bake in a 400°F. oven for 20 minutes. Serves 6.

POTATO PANCAKES

6 large potatoes
1 tablespoon CORNSTARCH
MILK
1 teaspoon salt
Pinch of baking powder
4 EGGS

Peel potatoes and soak for several hours in cold water. Grate, drain, and for every pint add 2 eggs, 1 tablespoon cornstarch dissolved in a little milk, ½ teaspoon salt and baking powder. Beat eggs well and mix with the rest of the ingredients. Drop by spoonfuls on a hot buttered frying pan in small cakes. Turn and brown other side. Serve 5 or 6.

Note: Maybe served with applesauce.

DESSERTS

Cakes

SOYALAC CAROB CUPCAKES

¼ cup corn-free shortening
½ cup cane, beet or brown sugar
2 EGG yolks
1 cup soya flour
1 teaspoon baking powder
2 tablespoons carob powder
½ cup Soyalac
⅓ cup water
1 teaspoon vanilla
2 EGG whites, beaten

Thoroughly cream shortening, sugar, and beaten egg yolks. Sift flour, baking powder, and carob powder together and add alternately with liquid to shortening. Add flavoring and beaten egg whites. Fill greased, medium cupcake pans two-thirds full and bake at 350°F. for 25 to 30 minutes, or until the tops spring back when lightly touched. Chocolate may be used if permitted. Makes 1 dozen.

POTATO FLOUR SPONGE

2 EGGS, separated
½ cup cane, beet or fruit sugar
½ teaspoon vanilla
2 tablespoons potato flour
½ teaspoon corn-free baking powder

Beat eggs separately. To yolks, beat sugar, vanilla, flour, and baking powder. Add stiffly beaten egg whites. Bake in a 350°F. oven in single layer tin for approximately 40 minutes. Serves 3 to 6.

QUICK DESSERT

Potato Flour Sponge*
Peaches
Whipped CREAM
Sherry or vanilla flavoring

Cut potato flour sponge with biscuit cutter. Place half a canned peach in center of sherbet glass. Cut biscuit in half, placing halves around peach (rounded side up) and using four pieces to each sherbet glass. Top peach with whipped cream, flavored with sherry or vanilla. Serves 4.

*See recipe above.

LEMON ICEBOX CAKE

1 layer Potato Flour Sponge, sliced in 4 to 6 pieces*
½ cup BUTTER
1 cup cane, beet or fruit sugar
4 EGGS, separated
Juice and grated rind of 1 lemon
¼ teaspoon salt
Whipped CREAM (optional)

Have ready potato flour sponge. Blend butter and sugar. Add yolks, lemon juice and rind. Add salt to egg whites and beat stiff (not dry). Fold in. Line mold with thin slices of Potato Flour Sponge, alternating with cream filling ½ inch thick. Cover with waxed paper. Chill for at least 6 hours. Serve with whipped cream (optional). Serves 4 to 6.

Note: Raisins may be added to filling.

*See recipe above.

PINEAPPLE UPSIDE-DOWN CAKE (See recipe Part 12)

CARROT CAKE (See recipe Part 13)

RICE CAKES (See recipe Part 13)

JELLY ROLL (See recipe Part 13)

SPONGE CAKES (See recipe Part 13)

CAROB ROLL (See recipe Part 13)

CAROB BROWNIES (See recipe Part 13)

NUT AND BUTTER CAKE (See recipe Part 13)

SPICE CAKE WITH PINEAPPLE ICING (See recipe Part 11)

PINEAPPLE ICING (See recipe Part 11)

WHITE CAKE WITH SOY FLOUR (See recipe Part 11)

SPICY SUGAR CAKE (See recipe Part 11)

BUTTERMILK CAKE

1 cup sugar
1 cup BUTTERMILK
1 teaspoon baking soda
6 tablespoons CORN OIL
1 teaspoon vanilla
2 cups rye FLOUR
½ cup rice FLOUR or CORNSTARCH
1 teaspoon cinnamon
1 teaspoon nutmeg
⅓ teaspoon ground cloves
1 cup seedless raisins

Mix sugar, buttermilk, soda and corn oil. Add vanilla. Add rye flour and rice flour (or cornstarch), sifted together, and remaining ingredients. Pour into a greased oblong pan. Bake in a 400°F. oven for about 45 minutes, or until brown. Serves 6 to 8.

ICEBOX CHEESE CAKE

1 EGG, separated
½ cup cold water
¼ teaspoon salt
1 envelope gelatin
1 cup cottage CHEESE
Juice and grated rind of ½ lemon
½ cup whipped CREAM
1 cup crushed CORNFLAKES
¼ cup BUTTER, melted
2 tablespoons sugar
½ tablespoon cinnamon

Slightly beat egg yolk. Add ¼ cup of the cold water and salt. Cook over boiling water until a custard consistency. Pour remaining ¼ cup cold water in bowl and sprinkle in gelatin. Add to hot custard, stirring until gelatin is dissolved. Add cottage cheese, lemon juice, and rind. Cool. When mixture begins to thicken, fold in whipped cream and stiffly beaten egg white. Mix cornflakes with butter, sugar and cinnamon. Line a springform pan. Add cheese mixture. Chill in refrigerator. Serves 6 to 8.

GINGERBREAD

2 cups soybean FLOUR
½ cup CORNSTARCH
1½ teaspoons baking soda
1 teaspoon cinnamon
1 teaspoon ginger
½ teaspoon cloves
½ teaspoon salt
½ cup sugar
½ cup BUTTER
1 EGG
1 cup molasses
1 cup hot water

Sift flour and cornstarch. Sift separately remaining dry ingredients. Blend sugar and butter. Mix in remaining ingredients in order given. Put in greased pan lined with greased paper. Bake in a preheated 350°F. oven for 35 minutes. Serves 5 or 6.

JAM CAKE

- 1½ cups soybean FLOUR
- ½ cup CORNSTARCH
- 1 cup sugar
- ⅓ cup BUTTER
- ½ cup BUTTERMILK
- 1 teaspoon baking powder
- 1 teaspoon cinnamon
- 1 cup jam (any kind)
- ½ teaspoon nutmeg
- ½ teaspoon baking soda
- 3 EGG yolks, beaten
- 3 EGG whites, beaten
- ½ teaspoon cloves
- ½ cup seedless raisins
- Whipping CREAM

Sift together flour and cornstarch. Blend sugar and butter. Mix in order given. Bake in moderate oven at 350°F. in loaf or layers for 45 minutes. Quantity can be doubled. Serves 8 to 10.

CHOCOLATE BUNDT CAKE

- ¼ cup BUTTER
- ¼ cup sugar
- Pinch of salt
- Grated rind of ½ lemon
- ½ cake yeast
- ½ cup SOUR CREAM
- 1 ounce sweet chocolate, melted
- 2 cups potato flour
- 1 cup rye FLOUR

Cream butter, sugar, and salt. Add lemon rind, yeast dissolved in sour cream, chocolate and flours. Cover with waxed paper and refrigerate. Grease a bundt pan and pour in batter. Bake at 400°F. for 1 hour. Serves 6 to 7.

CHOCOLATE FUDGE CAKE

- 2 tablespoons soybean FLOUR
- 1 tablespoon CORN-STARCH
- 1 cup sugar
- 3 ounces unsweetened chocolate or 6 tablespoons cocoa
- 1 tablespoon vanilla
- 2 EGGS
- ½ cup BUTTER, melted

Sift together flour and cornstarch. Add remaining ingredients, mixing well. Pour into a biscuit pan, spreading ¾ inch thick, and bake at 425°F. for 25 to 30 minutes. Serves 8 to 10.

CHOCOLATE ICEBOX CAKE

2 ounces German sweet chocolate
2 to 3 tablespoons cool water
4 EGGS, separated
Potato Flour Sponge*
Whipped CREAM

Melt chocolate over boiling water. Beat in egg yolks and vanilla. Beat egg whites until stiff and fold in. Line 6-cup mold with sliced potato flour sponge. Fill with mixture and chill 2 to 3 hours. Unmold and serve with whipped cream. Serves 6 to 8.

*See recipe this part.

CHOCOLATE CAKE LEAH

6 EGGS, separated
1 cup sugar
½ cup cocoa
Whipped CREAM

Blend egg yolks and sugar, then add cocoa. Beat egg whites until stiff and fold in. Pour into a 10x15-inch pan that has been lined with waxed paper buttered on both sides. Bake in a preheated 350°F. oven for about 15 minutes. Spread with whipped cream and roll on damp towel. Turn on flat platter and cover with whipped cream. Serves 6 to 8.

Note: Baking too long dries this cake out.

COCOA CUPCAKES

3 tablespoons fat
1 cup sugar
1 EGG, well beaten
½ cup MILK
1 cup barley flour
½ cup rice FLOUR
2 teaspoons baking powder
⅛ teaspoon salt
⅓ cup cocoa
1 teaspoon vanilla

Cream fat and sugar, then add egg and milk. Sift flours, baking powder and salt. Add to mixture with cocoa. Add vanilla. Bake in well greased muffin tins in preheated 425°F. oven for 15 minutes. Makes 8 to 10, depending on size.

QUICK COFFEE CAKE

¾ cup rye FLOUR
¼ cup CORNSTARCH
2 teaspoons baking powder
2 tablespoons BUTTER
¾ cup sugar
1 EGG
½ cup MILK
½ teaspoon vanilla
Brown sugar

Sift flour, cornstarch and baking powder together. Blend butter and sugar. Add remaining ingredients. Pour into greased baking pan. Cover with dots of butter and brown sugar. Bake in a 350°F. oven for 20 to 30 minutes, or until brown. Serves 3 to 4.

Note: This base may be used for fruit coffee cakes. Fresh peaches, blueberries, blue plums and sweet bing cherries are suitable fruits.

QUICK SOUR CREAM-YEAST COFFEE CAKE

½ cup sweet BUTTER
½ cup granulated sugar
Pinch of salt
Grated lemon rind of 1 lemon
2 EGGS
1 cake yeast
1 cup SOUR CREAM
1 cup potato flour
2 cups rye FLOUR
Additional BUTTER
¼ cup brown sugar
¼ cup nuts
¼ cup raisins or citron
2 ounces sweet chocolate (optional)

Blend butter and granulated sugar. Add salt and lemon rind. Beat in eggs, one at a time. Crumble yeast in sour cream and add to mixture. Add flours, combined and sifted two or three times. Cover with waxed paper and refrigerate. Roll dough, cover with butter, brown sugar, nuts, raisins or citron. Let stand 30 minutes. Bake in a 425°F. oven for 30 minutes, or until golden brown. Serves 6 to 8.

Note: For chocolate cake, melt sweet chocolate and add. Roll. Serves 8 to 12.

MAPLE SPONGE

2 envelopes gelatin
½ cup cold water
2 cups brown sugar
½ cup hot water
2 EGG whites, stiffly beaten
1 cup chopped nuts
Whipped CREAM

Soak gelatin in cold water for about 5 minutes. Put brown sugar and hot water in saucepan and bring to boiling point. Let boil for 10 minutes. Pour syrup gradually into gelatin and cool. When nearly set, add egg whites and nuts. Turn into a wet mold and chill. Serve with whipped cream. Serves 4.

PEACH UPSIDE-DOWN CAKE

1 cup rye FLOUR
1 tablespoon CORN-STARCH
2 teaspoons baking powder
½ teaspoon salt
1 cup granulated sugar
½ cup BUTTER, melted
3 EGGS, separated
½ cup peach juice
1 teaspoon vanilla
½ cup brown sugar
3½ cups canned peaches

Sift flour, cornstarch, baking powder and salt together. Cream granulated sugar and ¼ cup butter; Reserve ¼ cup butter for topping. Add egg yolks and peach juice. Add sifted dry ingredients. Stiffly beat egg whites and fold in with vanilla. Arrange melted butter, brown sugar, and peaches in bottom of baking dish and pour batter on top. Bake in 450°F. oven for 45 minutes. Cool slightly and turn out onto rack. Serves 6 or 7.

UPSIDE-DOWN CAKE

½ cup brown sugar
1 tablespoon BUTTER
4 slices pineapple OR 4 halves peaches, sliced
4 EGGS, separated
¾ cup granulated sugar
Grated rind and juice of ½ lemon
¾ cup potato flour
1 teaspoon baking powder

Melt brown sugar and butter in an ovenproof frying pan. Add pineapple or peaches. Beat egg yolks and granulated sugar. Add lemon rind and juice and continue beating. Stiffly beat egg whites and fold in. Combine flour and baking powder and add to batter. Pour into frying pan over fruit. Bake in a 350°F. moderate oven for 30 minutes. When done, turn out on a platter, with fruit side up. Serves 6 to 8.

Frostings

CHOCOLATE BOILED ICING

2¼ cups sugar
1 teaspoon light CORN SYRUP
1 cup boiling water
3 EGG whites, stiffly beaten
4 squares unsweetened chocolate

Combine sugar, syrup, and water. Place over low heat and stir constantly until sugar is dissolved and mixture boils. Continue cooking until a small amount of syrup forms a soft ball in cold water, or spins a long thread when dropped from tip of spoon. Pour syrup in fine stream over egg whites, beating constantly. Fold in chocolate, melted and cooled. Continue beating until stiff enough to spread on cake.

CREAMY CAROB ICING

½ cake carob
¾ cup MILK
½ cup cane, beet or fruit sugar
1 heaping teaspoon arrowroot

Melt carob. Add milk and sugar and bring to a boil. Add arrowroot dissolved in a little milk when boiling, stirring constantly. When thick remove from heat. Beat until cool. Makes 1¼ cups.

Candy

PUFFED RICE CANDY

⅓ cup brown sugar
1 cup granulated sugar
1 cup water
1 teaspoon vanilla
¼ teaspoon salt
4 cups puffed rice*

Cook sugars and water until it forms hard ball in cold water. Add vanilla and salt. Pour over puffed rice. Stir until rice is evenly coated. Turn into greased tin and cut into squares. Makes 2½ to 3 dozen, depending on size.

*This is a good substitute for nuts in flavor.

Cookies

TEA WAFERS

3 EGG whites, unbeaten
4 tablespoons cane, beet or fruit sugar
3 tablespoons rice FLOUR
4½ teaspoons soy butter, softened

Combine in order listed. Drop about 2 to 3 inches apart on a greased cookie sheet. Bake about 10 minutes in a 375°F. moderate oven until light brown around edges. Roll into tight rolls:

while still hot. They will remain in shape if they are cooled at once. Makes about 15.

CHOCOLATE MACAROONS

1 pound almonds
2 ounces Baker's chocolate
1 pound confectioners' cane, beet or fruit sugar, sifted
2 level teaspoons arrowroot
8 EGG whites, beaten

Mince almonds very fine. Grate chocolate, add sugar, arrowroot and egg whites. Drop batter by teaspoonfuls in damp hand. Roll. Drop on buttered baking sheet. Bake in a preheated 425°F. oven for 15 to 20 minutes, or until slight crust forms. Allow to cool before removing from pan. Makes about 3 dozen.

MACAROONS

1 EGG
½ cup cane, beet or fruit sugar
¼ teaspoon vanilla
⅔ cup rolled oats
Pinch of salt
⅓ cup chopped walnuts
2 teaspoons BUTTER, melted

Beat egg until very light. Add sugar slowly, beating constantly. And vanilla, oats, salt, nuts and butter. Drop by teaspoonfuls onto a greased baking sheet. Bake for 10 minutes in 350°F. oven. Remove from pan while warm. Makes 18.

OATMEAL COOKIES

- **1 tablespoons BUTTER**
- **2 cups brown cane, beet or fruit sugar**
- **1¾ cups rolled oats**
- **1 teaspoon corn-free baking powder**
- **¼ teaspoon salt**
- **2 EGGS**
- **½ teaspoon vanilla**

Cream butter and sugar together. Add remaining ingredients. Mix well. Drop in small portions leaving space for cookies to spread, on large baking sheet. Bake in a 400°F. oven for about 10 minutes. Makes about 2½ dozen.

ICEBOX COOKIES (See recipe Part 6)

ALMOND COOKIES

- **¾ cup almonds**
- **2 tablespoons cold water**
- **1 tablespoon vinegar**
- **5 EGGS, separated**
- **⅓ teaspoon corn-free baking powder**
- **4 tablespoons corn-free fat, melted**
- **Salt**

Blanch almonds. Bake until light brown, then put through almond grater. Place in strainer and pour over cold water mixed with vinegar. Drain. Dry in oven. Grind again. Beat egg yolks until thick and lemon colored. Add to almonds with fat, baking powder and salt. Stiffly beat egg whites and fold in. Fill greased gem pan two-thirds full. Bake for 25 minutes in a 250°F.—275°F. slow oven. Makes 9 large cookies.

ALMOND MACAROONS

1 cup Almond Macaroon Paste*
¾ cup cane, beet or fruit sugar
¼ teaspoon salt
3 EGG whites

Rub paste smooth. Work in sugar, then salt. Beat egg whites, one at a time, into paste. Let stand for 20 minutes. Shape mixture with pastry bag on ungreased paper-covered baking sheet. Shake damp cloth over tops to moisten. Bake at 300°F. for 30 minutes, or until surface is dry. Remove from paper when slightly cool. Store in a cool place overnight. Makes 2 dozen.

*See Almond Paste for Macaroons, Part 7.

DATE PECAN PUFFS

2 EGG whites
⅛ teaspoon cream of tartar
6 tablespoons cane, beet or fruit sugar
Vanilla
1 cup chopped dates
1 cup chopped nuts
Soy oil for greasing cake tins
Potato flour

Beat egg whites stiff. Add cream of tartar and beat again. Add 4 tablespoons of the sugar. Beat mixture (it should stand in peaks). Add remaining 2 tablespoons sugar. Fold. Add a few drops vanilla. Add dates and nuts. Drop on soy oil greased tin, dusted with potato flour. Bake in a preheated 250°F. oven for 25 to 30 minutes. Makes 18, depending on size.

DATE AND WALNUT DROPS (See recipe Part 7)

OATMEAL COOKIES, NO. 1 (See recipe Part 11)

OATMEAL COOKIES, NO. 2 (See recipe Part 11)

SOYALAC NUT CRESCENTS (See recipe Part 11)

CINNAMON STICKS (See recipe Part 14)

COCONUT MACAROONS (See recipe Part 14)

BILL'S DATE COOKIES (See recipe Part 14)

SHREWSBURY WAFERS (See recipe Part 14)

SOYBEAN COOKIES

6 EGGS, separated
1 cup cane, beet or fruit sugar
½ cup CREAM
½ cup soybean FLOUR
2 teaspoons baking powder
½ cup ground blanched almonds
½ cup ground walnuts
Grated rind of 1 lemon
½ teaspoon cinnamon
1 teaspoon vanilla
Pinch of salt

Beat egg whites until stiff. Beat egg yolks and sugar well. Add cream, flour, baking powder, nuts, lemon, cinnamon, vanilla, salt and egg whites. Bake in two shallow pans for 15 to 16 minutes in a 375°F. oven. Cut into 1x5-inch strips. Makes about 3½ to 4 dozen, depending on size.

PEANUT BUTTER COOKIES

1 cup soybean FLOUR
¼ cup CORNSTARCH
¼ teaspoon salt
¾ teaspoon soda
1 teaspoon baking powder
½ cup granulated sugar
½ cup brown sugar
1 EGG
½ cup shortening
½ cup peanut butter

Sift flour and cornstarch. Add remaining dry ingredients, shortening, egg, and peanut butter. Mix well. Drop on buttered cookie sheets. Bake in a 375°F. oven for 10 to 12 minutes. Makes 4 dozen.

"SNAILS" OR "SCHNECKEN"

¼ cup BUTTER
¼ cup sugar
Pinch of salt
1 EGG
Grated rind of ½ lemon
½ cup SOUR CREAM
1 cake yeast
½ cup potato flour or CORNSTARCH
Brown sugar
Nuts
Raisins

Blend butter, sugar and salt. Add egg, lemon rind, sour cream in which yeast is dissolved, and sifted flour or cornstarch. Cover with waxed paper and refrigerate. Roll in sheet and cover with butter and brown sugar, nuts, raisins. Roll sheet lengthwise and cut roll in 2-inch strips. Place in muffin tins, buttered and lined with brown sugar, nuts and raisins. Let rise 4 hours at 80°F. Bake in a preheated 450°F. oven for about 30 minutes. Makes 8.

Pies

PUMPKIN PIE

BUTTER
16 marshmallows
2 cups cooked pumpkin
⅔ cup cane or beet brown sugar
1 teaspoon salt
1½ teaspoon ginger (optional)
1 teaspoon cinnamon (optional)
2 tablespoons boiling water
8 rye crackers, crumbled (or rice flakes)
4 tablespoons orange juice or rum
4 EGG yolks
1½ cups whipping CREAM

Grease a 9-inch pie plate with butter. Sprinkle over with rye cracker crumbs (or rice flakes). Bake crust in hot oven 450°F. 10 or 15 minutes until light brown. Melt marshmallows over hot water. Add pumpkin, brown sugar and salt. Mix ginger and cinnamon with boiling water and add with orange juice, to melted mixture. When marshmallows are completely melted, remove from heat and add eggs. Beat until smooth. Chill in tray. Whip cream and fold in mixture. Put in tray. Freeze without stirring. Spread in pie shell before serving. Makes 6 or 8 servings.

BUTTERSCOTCH FILLING FOR PIE

1½ cups brown sugar
3 tablespoons CORNSTARCH
⅛ teaspoon salt
3 EGG yolks
1½ cups MILK
1½ tablespoons BUTTER
1 teaspoon vanilla
3 EGG whites, stiffly beaten

Mix sugar, cornstarch, and salt. Add egg yolks, milk and butter. Cook in the top of a double boiler, stirring until thick. Cool a little. Add vanilla. Pour into springform pan lined with crust (see recipe under Pie Crusts). Cover with meringue. Brown in a 300°F. oven for 35 to 40 minutes. Serves 5 to 6.

SPRINGFORM PIE CRUST

Swedish bread brumbs or rye wafer crumbs
1 tablespoon cane, beet, or sugar
¼ teaspoon cinnamon

Grease a springform pan with corn-free fat. Spread with finely rolled Swedish rye bread crumbs or rye wafer crumbs. Season with sugar and cinnamon. Brown in moderate 375°F. oven for 10 to 12 minutes. Makes 1 crust.

RYE CRACKER CRUST (See recipe Part 6)

RICE FLOUR PASTRY

2 tablespoons soy shortening
¾ cup rice FLOUR
Pinch of salt
¼ cup water

Blend shortening and flour with fingers. Add salt and water, blending with a spoon. Press evenly into a tart shell. Add filling. Bake in a 350°F. oven for 10 to 12 minutes, or until tender. Makes 3 tarts about 3 inches across.

BARLEY FLOUR PIE CRUST

1½ cups Cellu barley flour
½ teaspoon salt
1 teaspoon Cellu baking powder
4 tablespoons soy shortening
3 or 4 tablespoons water
Favorite fruit filling

Sift flour, salt and baking powder, then cut in shortening. Add enough water to make a stiff dough. Roll on floured board. If to be used for pastry shell, line pie pan. Bake at 400°F. for 10 to 15 minutes. Makes 1 crust. Double recipe for a two-crust pie. Fill with favorite filling.

SOY GRITS PIE CRUST

½ cup Cellu grainless mix
¼ cup Cellu soy grits
1 teaspoon sugar
¼ cup Cellu evaporated goat's MILK

Combine all ingredients in mixing bowl. Work for short while in hands to form smooth ball. Roll, or press into shape, on small 4½-inch individual pie tin. Bake in a preheated 325°F. oven for about 15 minutes. Makes 2 small pie shells.

PIE CRUST, NO. 1

2 tablespoons fat
1 cup Cellu wheatless mix
2½ tablespoons ice water

Cut fat into flour mixture with two knives until mixture resembles a coarse meal. Add just enough ice water to form stiff dough. Roll on lightly floured board to desired size. Bake in a 400°F. to 425°F. oven for 8 to 10 minutes. Makes 1 crust.

PIE CRUST, NO. 2

1 cup Soya carob flour
¼ teaspoon salt
½ cup corn-free shortening
3 to 4 tablespoons water

Mix flour and salt together. Mix in shortening using fingers or a fork. Add water. Mix lightly to make a ball. Roll out. Makes 1 9-inch crust (for two-crust pie double recipe).

PIE CRUST, NO. 3

¾ cup rye FLOUR
¼ cup CORNSTARCH
½ teaspoon salt
⅓ cup shortening
2 or 3 tablespoons ice water

Sift flour once before measuring. Sift flour, cornstarch and salt together. Cut in shortening with two knives, leaving some of the shortening in lumps the size of peas. Sprinkle ice water in lightly, a little at a time, over flour and shortening. At first blend in lightly with a fork, then gather dough together lightly with fingertips. Roll to fit pan. Bake in a 450°F. oven for 10 to 12 minutes. Use for fruit pies.

Puddings

ARROWROOT DESSERT

Potato flour sponge*
1 package arrowroot dessert
2 cups MILK
1 EGG, well beaten
¼ teaspoon almond extract
Whipped CREAM (optional)
Nuts (optional)

Make potato flour sponge ahead of time. Mix dessert and milk together in top of double boiler. Cook for 8 minutes, stirring constantly until thickened. Add egg during last 2 minutes of cooking. Flavor with almond extract. Line sherbet glasses with potato flour sponge slices. Pour in dessert and top with whipped cream and chopped nuts. Serves 4 to 6.

*See recipe under Cakes, this part.

BANANA SCOTCH

½ cup dark CORN SYRUP
3 tablespoons BUTTER
½ cup sugar
½ cup CREAM
3 large bananas, sliced
Whipped CREAM (optional)

Cook syrup, butter, sugar and cream over low heat for 5 minutes, stirring occasionally. Pour over bananas. Serve plain or with whipped cream. Serves 6.

BLUEBERRY CRUMB PUDDING

1¼ cups CORNFLAKE crumbs
¼ teaspoon cinnamon
¼ cup sugar
2 tablespoons BUTTER, melted
1 cup cooked or canned blueberries
Whipped CREAM

Mix first four ingredients. Grease casserole, cover with half cornflake mixture. Pour blueberries on top of mixture. Sprinkle with other half of cornflake mixture. Bake in a 350°F. oven for 20 minutes. Serve warm with whipped cream. Serves 4 to 5.

RYE APPLE CHALET

- **1 EGG yolk**
- **¼ cup sugar**
- **3 rye wafers**
- **¼ teaspoon baking powder**
- **1 EGG white, beaten**
- **¼ teaspoon vanilla**
- **1 apple, chopped**
- **1 teaspoon raisins**
- **1 teaspoon shortening, melted**

Beat egg yolk with sugar. Add rye wafers, which have been soaked in water and water squeezed out. Add remaining ingredients in order listed. Grease an 8x8-inch pan. Bake ingredients in a 350°F. oven for 20 to 30 minutes. Serves 6.

Torte

CARROT PECAN TORTE

- **1 cup ground pecans**
- **1 cup cooked sieved carrots**
- **5 EGG yolks**
- **½ teaspoon grated lemon rind**
- **2 tablespoons potato flour**
- **5 EGG whites, stiffly beaten**
- **½ cup brown sugar, firmly packed**
- **1 teaspoon corn-free baking powder**
- **½ cup almonds**
- **1 cup whipped CREAM**

Mix pecans and carrots. Beat egg yolks until thick. Add sugar, baking powder, lemon juice and rind and beat until light and thick. Stir in carrots and pecans and flour. Fold in stiffly beaten egg whites. Grease springform. Bake at 300°F. for 1½ hours. When cool, will drop slightly in center. Cover with chopped almonds and whipped cream. Serves 4 or 5.

SAUCES AND GRAVIES

MUSHROOM SAUCE

½ pound fresh mushrooms, cleaned and chopped
1½ cups hot water
2 tablespoons arrowroot
2 tablespoons BUTTER
Salt

Sauté mushrooms in butter for 3 minutes. Add hot water and arrowroot blended with a little cold water. Cook 5 minutes more. Season with salt. Serve hot with steak or roast beef. Makes approximately 3 cups.

MEDIUM CREAM SAUCE WITH RICE FLOUR
(See recipe Part 13)

RYE FLOUR GRAVY (See recipe Part 13)

SECTION V

MISCELLANEOUS

INTRODUCTION

Truly one can be allergic to any of "100,000" things. In this 100,000 are the rest of the foods not detailed in the previous 15 parts of this book. Some of the foods are hardly allergenic at all, others are more so. Some of the more common offenders are discussed in this part.

Part 16 contains a list of food families and is included to assist in selecting foods less likely to cause allergy. If one finds himself highly allergic to mountain trout, he might well eat only a small piece of the next fish he tries until he see that it won't bother him. If he is highly allergic to many other things as well, he would better avoid all fish until he is under control. Actually among these food families there are only three groups where cross-reactions between members are of any great importance. These are: the cereal grains, legumes and the plum (prune) families. Even among these three, though, people can be highly allergic one member and eat the others with impunity. In any case it is always best to proceed with caution within a group when highly allergic to one member.

Part 17 consists of a number of foods not previously discussed and their role in the production of allergies.

Part 18 is entitled Baking Notes. Little difficulty is encountered in substituting one meat or vegetable for another but one flour for another in baking is a different matter. Wheat flour contains a "gluing together" substance that some other flours do not. Therefore, some practice may be required to turn out a most desirable product.

Part 19 is composed of a list of manufacturers of foods, recipes and literature on the subject of allergy.

Part 20 is the Index.

PART 16

Food Families

Amphibians
Frogs

Birds
Chicken
- Chicken eggs

Duck
- Duck eggs

Goose
- Goose eggs

Grouse
Guinea hen
- Guinea hen eggs

Partridge
Pheasant
Quail
Squab
Turkey

Crustaceans
Crab
Crayfish
Lobster
Shrimp

Mammals
Beef
Beef gelatin
Butter
Cow's milk
- Lactose

Veal
Goat
- Goat's milk
- Goat's milk cheese

Horse meat
Mutton
- Lamb

Pork
- Bacon
- Ham
- Lard
- Pork gelatin

Rabbit
Squirrel
Venison

Mollusks
Abalone
Clam
Mussel
Oyster
Squid

Reptiles
Rattlesnake
Turtle

Fish

Barracuda
Bass
Black bass
Bluefish
Buffalo
Bullhead
Butterfish
Carp
Catfish
Cod
  Scrod
Croaker
Cusk
Dru
Eel
Flounder
Haddock
Hake
Halibut
Harvestfish
Mullet
Muskellunge
Perch
Pickerel
Pike
Pollack
Pompano
Porgy
Rosefish
Scup
Snapper
Sole
Sucker
Sunfish
Swordfish
Tuna
Weakfish

Apple Family

Apple
Apple butter
Apple pectin
Cider
  Vinegar
Pear
Quince
  Quince seed

Arrowroot Family

Arrowroot

Arum Family

Dasheen
Taro
  Poi

Aster Family

Artichoke
Dandelion
Endive
Escarole
Celtuce
Head lettuce
Jerusalem artichoke
Leaf lettuce
Oyster plant
  Chicory
Sunflower seed oil

Banana Family

Banana
Plantain

Birch Family

Filbert
Hazelnut
Oil of birch
  Wintergreen

Brazil Nut Family

Brazil nut

Buckwheat Family
Buckwheat
Garden Sorrel
Rhubarb

Cactus Family
Prickly pear

Caltrap Family
Gum Guaiac

Caper Family
Capers

Cashew Family
Cashew
Mango
Pistachio

Cereal Family
Bamboo Shoots
Barley
  Malt
  Maltose
Cane
  Cane sugar
  Molasses
Corn
  Cornmeal
  Cornstarch
  "Kremel"
  Corn oil
  "Mazola"
Corn Sugar
  "Cerelose"
  "Dyno"
  Dextrose
Corn Syrup
  "Cartose"
  Glucose
  "Karo"
  "Puretose"
  "Sweetose"
Grits
  Hominy
  Millet
Oats
  Oatmeal
Rice
  Brown rice
Sorghum
  Kafir
Wheat
  Bran
  Farina
  Flour
  Gluten flour
  Graham flour
  Wheat Germ
  Whole-wheat flour
Wild rice

Citrus Family
Citron
Grapefruit
Kumquat
Lemon
Lime
Orange
Tangerine

Cochliospermum Family
Gum karaya

Ebony Family
Persimmon

Fungi Family
Mushroom
Yeast

Ginger Family
Cardamon
Ginger
Turmeric

Gooseberry Family

Currant
Gooseberry

Goosefoot Family

Beet
  Beet sugar
Chard
Lamb's quarters
Spinach

Gourd Family

Cantaloupe
Casaba
Christmas melon
Cucumber
Honeydew
Muskmelon
Persian melon
Pumpkin
Squash
Watermelon

Grape Family

Brandy
Champagne
Grape
  Cream of Tartar
Raisin
Wine
Wine vinegar

Heath Family

Blueberry
Cranberry
Huckleberry

Holly Family

Mate

Honeysuckle Family

Elderberry

Iris Family

Saffron

Laurel Family

Avocado
Bay Leaves
Cinnamon
Sassafras

Legume Family

Black-eyed pea
Carob
  St. John's Bread
Gum Acacia
Gum tragacanth
Jack bean
Licorice
Lima bean
Navy bean
Pea
Peanut
  Peanut oil
Soy Bean
Lecithin
Soybean flour
Soybean Oil
Tonka bean

Lily Family

Asparagus
Garlic
Onion

Madder Family

Coffee

Mallow Family

Cottonseed meal
  Cottonseed oil
Okra

Maple Family

Maple sugar
Maple syrup

Mint Family

Horehound
Marjoram
Mint
Peppermint
Sage
Savory
Spearmint
Thyme

Mulberry Family

Breadfruit
Fig
Hop
Mulberry

Mustard Family

Broccoli
Brussels sprouts
Cabbage
Cauliflower
Celery cabbage
Collard
Colza shoots
Horseradish
Kale
Kohlrabi
Mustard
  Mustard greens
Radish
Rutabaga
Turnip
Watercress

Myrtle Family

Allspice
Cloves
Guava
Pimiento

Nutmeg Family

Mace
Nutmeg

Oak Family

Chestnut

Olive Family

Green olive
Ripe olive
  Olive oil

Palm Family

Coconut
  Coconut oil
Date
Palm cabbage
Sago

Papaya Family

Papaya

Parsley Family

Angelica
Anise
Caraway
Celeriac
Coriander
Cumin
Dill
Fennel
Parsley
Parsnip
Water Celery

Papaw Family

Papaw

Pepper Family

Black pepper
White pepper

Pine Family

Juniper
Piñon nut

Pineapple Family

Pineapple

Plum Family
Almond
Apricot
Cherry
Nectarine
Peach
Plum
  Prune

Pomegranate Family
Pomegranate

Poppy Family
Poppyseed

Potato Family
Chili
Eggplant
Green pepper
Ground cherry
Potato
Red pepper
  Capsicum
  Cayenne
Tobacco
Tomato

Purslane Family
New Zealand spinach
Purslane

Rose Family
Blackberry
Black raspberry
Boysenberry
Dewberry
Loganberry
Red raspberry
Strawberry
Youngberry

Sapodilla
Chicle

Sesame Family
Sesame oil

Soapberry Family
Litchi

Spurge Family
Jassava Meal
Tapioca

Stercula Family
Cocoa
Chocolate
Cocoa butter
Cola beans

Sweet Potato Family
Sweet potato

Tea Family
Tea

Walnut Family
Black walnut
Butternut
English walnut
Hickory nut
  Pecan

Yam Family
Chinese potato
Yam

PART 17

More Allergic Foods

1. CHOCOLATE:
Chocolate is both an allergen and an ephithelial stimulant. In the latter role chocolate or cocoa may be bad for acne. It is not sugar or candy that is bad for the skin—it is the chocolate. Carob is rapidly becoming a welcome substitute for chocolate. Several carob recipes can be found in the text.
2. COFFEE:
Coffee may cause allergy although commonly the "allergy" may be the stimulation caused by caffeine. If stimulation is the problem, caffeine-free coffees may be used. Otherwise, there are cereal grain substitutes such as the time-honored "Postum"!
3. COTTONSEED:
There are not many cases of allergy to cottonseed but we are seeing more and more each year in testing for allergies. Cottonseed allergies may bc severe and are, as usual found in ingestants, inhalants and contactants. Cottonseed meal is used for fertilizer and animal food and as such may appear in cow's milk. The flour is used for human food, and in gins and soft drinks. The oil is used for foods such as cooking oils, salad oils, shortenings, mayonnaise, sardines, commercial frying and baking, candy and ointments. It is used in the manufacture of many things including paper, paint and cosmetics.

Pure long-fiber cotton such as used in men's shirts, contains no cottonseed. Linters, the short fiber remaining on the seeds, do contain fragments of seeds and can cause both contact and inhalation allergies since they are used in cotton batting or wadding for all kinds of cushions, pads, mattresses and upholstering.

4. FLAXSEED:
Flaxseed is used in almost the same way as cottonseed, although less in food products. Flaxseed is a rare but potent allergen. Allergies have occurred from milk of cows fed flax and from linen clothing as well as by inhalation of fumes of products containing flax.

5. FRUITS:
There are many different families of fruits so there will likely be no problem supplying several for the diet. In particular, fruits of the rose family seem to cause the most trouble.

6. GREENS:
Perhaps surprisingly many people are allergic to lettuce and cabbage, and fewer to spinach. In such cases other greens have been used with success, particularly beet, turnip, kale and dandelion greens or watercress. If not allergic to parsley, it is a good food for roughage, vitamins and minerals.

7. KARAYA GUM:
This gum is a substitute for acacia and tragacanth gums and as such is used in many foods and drugs. Ever wonder why your cherry pie flows into the space left after a piece is removed and the store bought pie doesn't? Cookies, candies, hand lotions, toothpastes and some gelatins are among the users of gums.

8. MEATS:

8a FISH:
Reactions to true (vertebrate) fish are not common, but the allergy may be very severe. Cross-reactions are not common either so another fish may be tried in small amounts.

8b MAMMALS:
The meats of the mammals are easily recognized. Other areas of contact include gelatin often made from beef and pork. Veal may be used with chicken in salads. Oftentimes allergy to hog products may be caused by the food the animal eats. Bacon drippings are recognizable, but animal fats and oils may be disguised beef or pork derivatives. Lamb and mutton cause much less allergy. A gelatin substitute is agar-agar. The widespread use of beef probably makes it the leading allergy offender of the meats.

8c POULTRY:
Cross-sensitivity between the various birds is rare because they are not very close genetically. The eggs of the various birds, however, are very close—allergy to one almost always implies allergy to another. The use of antibiotics and hormones in bird feeding can lead to reactions in a few people.

8d SHELLFISH:
The two families of edible shellfish, crustaceans and mollusks, are by no means even closely related to each other nor to vertebrate fish. Because one is allergic to shrimp he should not think himself to be automatically allergic to clams or sea bass.

9. NUTS:
Nuts bother few people but when they do, the reactions may be severe. It seems everyone knows of someone whose mouth swells from a bit of cake with a pecan in it. Again, cross-reaction is not common so do not give up the flavor of all nuts because of one or two. Crisped cereals can often replace nuts in a recipe.

10. POTATOES:
The potato family includes two of the more evident food allergies, the white potato and the tomato. Potatoes are rather low in both frequency and severity considering their widespread use. Tomato is low in frequency but more severe in its effects, especially as it affects the skin. This family also includes one of the horrors of the world—tobacco.

11. SPICES:
Spices cause gastrointestinal upsets because they are indigestible. What pepper does to the nose so does it do to the whole digestive tract—irritates it. If a true allergy occurs, fruit juice concentrates and some flavoring extracts can be used.

12. SUGAR:
Sugar is the gasoline of the body, carbohydrates are reduced to glucose to burn for energy. If one is "allergic" to sugar it is because he is very, very sensitive to that from which sugar is derived whether corn, beet, cane or fruit, and more usually corn. The amounts of corn or beet or cane or fruit in refined sugar is miniscule in amount, unless, as in confectioners' sugar, cornstarch is added. As a substitute for sugar, various honeys may be tried but one can be allergic to the flowers from which honey is derived.

13. TAPIOCA:
Tapioca is a good substitute for other foods, particularly in the flour form. If allergic to tapioca, however, one must be careful with yeast and choose a yeast without a tapioca base or use baking powder in place of yeast. To thicken sauces a cereal grain can be used.

14. TEA:
Tea is a gastrointestinal irritant as is coffee. True allergy can occur, in which case maté or Kaffir tea may be substituted.
15. VEGETABLES:
Vegetables rarely cause severe allergic reactions—although the legumes are always a suspect in food allergy and are more capable of cross-sensitivity. When highly allergic to peanuts one must be careful with soybean as a substitute for milk. People may eructate (burp) after eating cucumber but this is not truly an allergy. Soybeans have been known in Asia for centuries but in the U.S.A. only since the end of the 18th century. Soy is now found in "everything"; cereals, breads, sauces, candies, meats, salad dressings, milk substitutes, ice cream, soups, and even as vegetable sprouts. Soy is used extensively in industry also; paints, linoleum, blankets, cosmetics, soaps, fertilizer, illuminating oil, gearshift knobs—you name it!

A good substitute for onion and garlic is green pepper or green pimiento.

Insect sprays on fruits and vegetables occasionally cause trouble.

PART 18

Baking Notes

Baking encompasses particularly the use of GRAINS, MILK, EGGS, SHORTENINGS and BAKING POWDER. There are many pure grains on the market manufactured by reliable companies (see Part 19), good soy substitutes for milk, shortenings free of substances to which you may be allergic and ways to avoid the use of eggs and baking powders, if necessary. This book contains recipes using all possible combinations of allergenic foods so that a complete diet can be maintained including all the "goodies" anyone could desire. We have capitalized the four "offenders" in each chapter as an alert if you are allergic to these ingredients.

GRAINS:

WHEAT and CORN are the most common grains used in baking and the ones which cause the most allergy also. In many cases of allergy substitutes have to be used. If the person is highly allergic it might be best to try little-used flours such as arrowroot for a starter.

A list of replacements for wheat flour follows:

For 1 cup of wheat flour you may substitute:

½ cup arrowroot
½ cup barley
¾ cup buckwheat flour
1 cup corn flour

¾ cup cornmeal (coarse)
1 scant cup cornmeal (fine)
½ cup cornstarch
¾ cup oats
1⅓ to 1½ cups oats (ground rolled)
¾ cup potato meal
⅝ cup potato starch
¾ to ⅞ cup rice flour
¾ to 1 cup rye flour
1 cup rye meal
¾ cup soybean flour
1 cup purified wheat starch
½ cup potato flour and ½ cup rye flour
⅓ cup potato flour and ⅔ cup rye flour
½ cup potato starch flour and ½ cup soy flour
⅝ cup rice flour and ⅓ cup rye flour
1 cup soy flour and ¼ cup potato starch flour

NOTES:

A combination of flours is often more palatable than a single flour. Combinations should be sifted together three times to ensure good mixing and then thoroughly mixed with other dry ingredients. Baking time is usually longer with flours other than wheat by perhaps 10 to 20 minutes, especially when milk and eggs are omitted from the recipe. A lower baking temperature is also better.

Do not be concerned if batters appear thinner or thicker than usual wheat flour batters.

Refrigerating dough mixture for 30 minutes makes the dough easier to handle and improves the appearance of the final product.

Cakes made from other than wheat flours are likely to be drier. Frosting plus storing in a closed container will help. Fruits, chocolate chips and nuts added to cakes will improve the texture.

Muffins and biscuits made from non-wheat flours have a better texture when made small.

Arrowroot flour may be used one-for-one for Cornstarch.

Cornmeal products have grainy textures. If Cornmeal is cooked or scalded after measuring a smoother texture will result. One tablespoon of cornstarch may be used to thicken ½ cup of custard instead of wheat. Corn flour is a smooth flour that can be blended with other flours for baking.

Oat flours are grainy and are better scalded after measuring and before using.

Potato flour has become increasingly popular over the years but has its allergy-causing powers, also. It is best as a basis for sponge cake. Potato starch flour is close textured and very white and will generally be used. Potato meal is grainy, although less so than cornmeal, and used in small amounts can lighten the texture of a bread. Potato meal makes excellent breading for meats, fish, and fowl. Potato water, saved after boiling potatoes, makes bread lighter than plain water.

Rice products have grainy textures also. In many instances Rice flour can be mixed with the liquid(s) in the recipe, boiled and then cooled before being added to the other ingredients. Rice flakes makes good breading for meats, fish and fowl.

Rye bread must be kneaded thoroughly and raised carefully.

Soy flour simply cannot be used alone because of its oiliness and unusual flavor. It has been used satisfactorily in combinations, particularly with Potato flour.

Tapioca flour is used more sparingly even in thickening gravies and sauces or they will become gummy.* One-half teaspoon in a small amount of cold water will thicken 1 cup of hot liquid. Fruit pies may be thickened with 1 tablespoon. TAPIOCA is not a good flour to use for cakes and cookies.

Taro meal makes interesting piecrusts.

Other flours such as barley, buckwheat, and lima bean may be experimented with, also.

*Excellent thickening agent where small amounts are needed are: Lecithinated CORN Flour, Lecithinated Soya Flour and Lecithinated WHEAT Flour, as the case may be.

MILK:

Substitution of cow's MILK in cooking has been made easier over the years by using soybean preparations. Many of these require sugar or salt to taste. In many recipes plain water or coconut milk can be used. A number of people will find goat's milk satisfactory but remember its casein fraction is the same as that in cow's MILK. There are milkless "whipped creams" in pressure cans to top off a custard. Basic cream sauce directions are found under Sauces in Part 13.

EGGS:

When EGGS are to be omitted from a recipe for batter or dough an extra teaspoon of egg-free baking powder will have to be used to replace each egg. If cornstarch is allowed, 1 tablespoon can replace one egg in a custard. One tablespoon of a vegetable oil with 2 tablespoons of water may replace an egg in most recipes. Jolly Joan Egg Replacer can be used.

There is a new egg substitute available, Morningstar Farms, and it can be found in the frozen food section of your market.

SHORTENING:

Throughout these recipes the words fat and shortening are interchangeable in baking procedures. Whether it is runny or a solid doesn't matter. Oils for salads and cooking are the same. Whether the shortening is vegetable or animal depends upon your allergy and flavor requirements. Some shortenings contain MILK and/or EGGS such as margarines—be sure. Hydrogenated MILK-free fats are available. Bacon drippings, lamb drippings,

Recommended Dietary Allowances, Revised 1980*
Designed for the maintenance of good nutrition of practically all healthy people in the U.S.A.
FOOD AND NUTRITION BOARD, NATIONAL ACADEMY OF SCIENCES-NATIONAL RESEARCH COUNCIL

age and sex group	*weight*		*height*		*protein*	*fat-soluble vitamins*			*water soluble vitamins*		
	kg.	*lb.*	*cm.*	*in.*		*vitamin A*	*vitamin D*	*vitamin E*	*vitamin C*	*thiamin*	*riboflavin*
					gm.	*μg.R.E.†*	*μ.g.‡*	*mg.αT.E.#*	← *mg.*		→
infants											
0.0-0.5 yr.	6	13	60	24	kg.x2.2	420	10	3	35	0.3	0.4
0.5-1.0 yr.	9	20	71	28	kg.x2.0	400	10	4	35	0.5	0.6
children											
1-3 yr.	13	29	90	35	23	400	10	5	45	0.7	0.8
4-6 yr.	20	44	112	44	30	500	10	6	45	0.9	1.0
7-10 yr.	28	62	132	52	34	700	10	7	45	1.2	1.4
males											
11-14 yr.	45	99	157	62	45	1,000	10	8	50	1.4	1.6
15-18 yr.	66	145	176	69	56	1,000	10	10	60	1.4	1.7
19-22 yr.	70	154	177	70	56	1,000	7.5	10	60	1.5	1.7
23-50 yr.	70	154	178	70	56	1,000	5	10	60	1.4	1.6
51+yr.	70	154	178	70	56	1,000	5	10	60	1.2	1.4
females											
11-14 yr.	46	101	157	62	46	800	10	8	50	1.1	1.3
15-18 yr.	55	120	163	64	46	800	10	8	60	1.1	1.3
19-22 yr.	55	120	163	64	44	800	7.5	8	60	1.1	1.3
23-50 yr.	55	120	163	64	44	800	5	8	60	1.0	1.2
51+ yr.	55	120	163	64	44	800	5	8	60	1.0	1.2
pregnancy					+30	+200	+5	+2	+20	+0.4	+0.3
lactation					+20	+400	+5	+3	+40	+0.5	+0.5

*The allowances are intended to provide for individual variations among most normal persons as they live in the United States under usual environmental stresses. Diets should be based on a variety of common foods in order to provide other nutrients for which human requirements have been less well defined. See text for detailed discussion of allowances and of nutrients not tabulated. See preceding table for weights and heights of individual year of age and for suggested average energy intakes.
†Retinol equivalents; 1 retinol equivalent = 1μ.g. retinol or 6μ.g. β-carotene. See text for calculation of vitamin activity of diets as retinol equivalents.
‡As cholecalciferol: 10 μg. cholecalicferol = 400 I.U. vitamin D.
#αtocopherol equivalents: 1 mg. d-α-tocopherol = 1αT.E. See text for variation in allowances and calculation of vitamin E activity of the diet as α tocopherol equivalents.
¶1 N.E. (niacin equivalent) = 1 mg. niacin or 60 mg. dietary tryptophan.
||The folacin allowances refer to dietary sources as determined by *Lactobacillus casei*

water soluble vitamins				*minerals*					
niacin	*vitamin B_6*	*folacin‖*	*vitamin B_{12}*	*calcium*	*phosphorus*	*magnesium*	*iron*	*zinc*	*iodine*
mg.N.E.¶	*mg.*	← *μg.* →		←		*mg.*		→	*μg.*
6	0.3	30	0.5**	360	240	50	10	3	40
8	0.6	45	1.5	540	360	70	15	5	50
9	0.9	100	2.0	800	800	150	15	10	70
11	1.3	200	2.5	800	800	200	10	10	90
16	1.6	300	3.0	800	800	250	10	10	120
18	1.8	400	3.0	1,200	1,200	350	18	15	150
18	2.0	400	3.0	1,200	1,200	400	18	15	150
19	2.2	400	3.0	800	800	350	10	15	150
18	2.2.	400	3.0	800	800	350	10	15	150
16	2.2	400	3.0	800	800	350	10	15	150
15	1.8	400	3.0	1,200	1,200	300	18	15	150
14	2.0	400	3.0	1,200	1,200	300	18	15	150
14	2.0	400	3.0	800	800	300	18	15	150
13	2.0	400	3.0	800	800	300	18	15	150
13	2.0	400	3.0	800	800	300	10	15	150
+2	+0.6	+400	+1.0	+400	+400	+150	††	+5	+25
+5	+0.5	+100	+1.0	+400	+400	+150	††	+10	+50

assay after treatment with enzymes ("conjugases") to make polyglutamyl forms of the vitamin available to the test organism.

**The RDA for vitamin B_{12} in infants is based on average concentration of the vitamin in human milk. The allowances after weaning are based on energy intake (as recommended by the American Academy of Pediatrics) and consideration of other factors, such as intestinal absorption; see text.

††The increased requirement during pregnancy cannot be met by the iron content of habitual American diets or by the existing iron stores of many women; therefore, the use of 30 to 60 mg. supplemental iron is recommended. Iron needs during lactation are not substantially different from those of non-pregnant women, but continued supplementation of the mother for two to three months after parturition is advisable in order to replenish stores depleted by pregnancy.

Estimated safe and adequate daily dietary intakes of additional selected vitamins and minerals*

age group	*vitamins*			*trace elements†*		
	vitamin K	*biotin*	*pantothenic acid*	*copper*	*manganese*	*fluoride*
	← μg. →		←			→
infants						
0.0-0.5 yr.	12	35	2	0.5-0.7	0.5-0.7	0.1-0.5
0.5-1.0 yr.	10- 20	50	3	0.7-1.0	0.7-1.0	0.2-1.0
children and adolescents						
1-3yr.	15- 30	65	3	1.0-1.5	1.0-1.5	0.5-1.5
4-6 yr.	20- 40	85	3-4	1.5-2.0	1.5-2.0	1.0-2.5
7-10 yr.	30- 60	120	4-5	2.0-2.5	2.0-3.0	1.5-2.5
11+yr.	50-100	100-200	4-7	2.0-3.0	2.5-5.0	1.5-2.5
adults	70-140	100-200	4-7	2.0-3.0	2.5-5.0	1.5-4.0

*From Recommended Dietary Allowances, Revised 1980. Food and Nutrition Board, National Academy of Sciences—National Research Council. Because there is less information on which to base allowances, these figures are not given in the main table of RDAs and are provided here in the form of recommended intakes.

trace elements†			electrolytes		
chromium	selenium	molybdenum	sodium	potassium	chloride
← mg. →					
0.01-0.04	0.01-0.04	0.03-0.06	115- 350	350- 925	275- 700
0.02-0.06	0.02-0.06	0.04-0.08	250- 750	425-1,275	400-1,200
0.02-0.08	0.02-0.08	0.05-0.1	325- 975	550-1,650	500-1,500
0.03-0.12	0.03-0.12	0.06-0.15	450-1,350	775-2,325	700-2,100
0.05-0.2	0.05-0.2	0.1 -0.3	600-1,800	1,000-3,000	925-2,775
0.05-0.2	0.05-0.2	0.15-0.5	900-2,700	1,525-4,575	1,400-4,200
0.05-0.2	0.05-0.2	0.15-0.5	1,100-3,300	1,875-5,625	1,700-5,100

†Since the toxic levels for many trace elements may be only several times usual intakes, the upper levels for the trace elements given in this table should not be habitually exceeded.

chicken fat and rendered beef suet can all be used within one's allergy limits, each imparting its own flavor to the finished product.

BAKING POWDER:

Starch flours require more leavening than WHEAT, which has gluten to hold things together. When gluten is not present, the "flour" is not a flour, rather it is a starch. Even WHEAT can be rendered gluten-free—a starch. Many baking powders contain CORNSTARCH and EGG—read the label. A satisfactory leavening agent can be made egg-free; 1½ teaspoons of cream of tartar combined with ½ teaspoon of baking soda is equal to 1 teaspoon of baking powder.

SUGAR:

Fruit sugar is becoming very popular as a sugar substitute. One of these is fructose, which is used to replace ordinary sugar in cereals, cold drinks and desserts. Make sure you are not allergic to the fruit from which this product is derived.

You may omit salt and preferably use condiments as salt has been found to aggravate *some* allergies.

PART 19

Special Food Sources, Recipes and Literature

Your Drugstore
Your Grocery Market
Your Health Food Store
A I A Allergy Information Association, 3 Powburn Place, Weston, Ontario, Canada
Adolph's Ltd. (salt substitute) 5355 Cartwright Street, North Hollywood, Calif. 91601
Alba Foods (skim milk products), 800 Third Avenue, New York, N.Y. 10020
Alberto Culver Co. (Sugar Twin), Melrose Park, Ill. 60160
Akin Distributors, Inc. 8460 San Fernando Road, Sun Valley, Calif. 91352
Akin Distributors, Inc., P.O. Box 515, Jacksonville, Fla. 32201, OR Box 2658, Tulsa, Okla. 74101
Allergy Foundation of America, 801 Second Ave., N.Y., N.Y. 10017
American Dietetic Assn., 620 No. Michigan Ave., Chicago, Ill. 60611
American Lecithin Co. (Lecithinated wheat, soya, corn flours) 32-60 - 61st Street, Woodside, Long Island, N.Y. 11377
Balanced Foods, Inc., 700 Broadway, N.Y. 10003
Batter Lite Foods (fructose, batter lite cake batters, etc.) P.O. Box 321, Beloit, Wisc. 53511
Battle Creek Foods Co., Fourth St., Battle Creek, Mich. 49017
Beatrice Foods, 1526 So. State St., Chicago, Ill. 69605
Borden Co. (The) (Mull-Soy), 350 Madison Ave., N.Y., N.Y. 10017

Cal-Power Beverages, (Choco imitation whole egg powder), 4620 W. 77th St., Minneapolis, Minn. 55434

Campbell Soup Co., 375 Memorial Ave., Camden, N.Y. 08101

Carnation Foods (special ice creams and pastries), 14th & Poplar, Oakland, Calif. 94607

Clinical Research Unit, University of Michigan Medical Center, Ann Arbor, Mich. 48109

Chicago Dietetic Supply House (Cellu), 1750 Van Buren Street, Chicago, Ill. 69612

Chico Foods, Box 1004, Chico, Calif. 95926

Cumberland Packing Co. (Butter Buds), 1636 Taylor, Racine, Wisc. 53403

Cumberland Sugar Co. (Sweet 'n Low), 2 Cumberland Street, Brooklyn, N.Y. 11205

Diet & Health Products (Fisher Cheese Co.), P.O. Box 1886, Lima, Ohio 45802

El Molino Mills (carob, cereals, flours, mixes), P.O. Box 2025, Alhambra, Calif. 91803

Eli Lilly & Co., Indianapolis, Ind. 46206

Ener-G-Cereals, Inc. (Jolly Joan), 1526 Utah Ave. South, Seattle, Wash. 98134

Fearn Soya Foods Co. (Richard's Food Corp.), 4520 James Place, Melrose Park, Ill. 60160

Fisher Cheese Co. (count-down cheese products, milk free Cheezola), P.O. Box 12, Wapakoneta, Ohio 45995

Frito Lay, Inc. (Bakenets, pork rind snax), Exchange Park, P.O. Box 35034, Dallas, Tex. 75235

General Mills Chemical, Inc. (Yoplait), P.O. Box 1113, Minneapolis, Minn. 55440

Good Food Unit #306, National Health Systems, The Times, P.O. Box 1501, Ann Arbor, Mich. 48106

Haddon House Products (Jane's Krazy Mixed-up Salt), Marlton Pike, Medford, N.Y. 08055

Health Food Distributors, 7657 W. McNichols Road, Detroit, Mich. 48221

Health Food Jobbers, Inc., 216-226 North Clinton, Chicago, Ill. 60606

Holister-Stier, 2030 Wilshire Blvd., Los Angeles, Calif. 90057

Henkel Corp. (Dietary specialties), 4620 W. 7th St., Minneapolis, Minn. 55435

Kahan & Lessin Company, 2425 Hunter St., Los Angeles, Calif. 90021

Knox Gelatin (Thomas J. Lipton, Inc.) (salad dressings), 300 Sylvan Ave., Englewood Cliffs, N.J. 07632

Kraft Foods, 500 Peshtigo Court, Chicago, Ill. 69690

Lever Bros., Inc., New York, N.Y. 10022

Loma Linda Foods (Soyalac), Riverside, Calif. 92502

M C P Foods (Slimset, mix for jams and jellies), P.O. Box 3633, Anaheim, Calif. 92803

Mead Johnson & Co. (Sobee, Nutramigen), Evansville, Ind. 47708

National Dairy Council, 6300 No. River Road, Rosemont, Ill. 60018

National Health Systems, P.O. Box 1501, Ann Arbor, Mich. 48106

Nutri Books, 1523-B Nineteenth St., Denver, Col. 80202

Nu Vita Foods, 7524 SW Macadam Ave., Portland, Ore. 97219

Pillsbury Co. (Sprinkle Sweet), 311 - 2nd St. SE, Minneapolis, Minn. 55414

Plough, Inc. (Ril Sweet), Memphis, Tenn. 38101

Quaker Oats Co. (The), Merchandise Mart Plaza, Chicago, Ill. 60654

Ralston Purina Co., Checkerboard Square, St. Louis, Mo. 63199

Richard's Foods Corp., 4520 James Place, Melrose Park, Ill. 60160

Roger Brothers, Twin Falls, Idaho 83301

Rosarita Foods Products (Mexican foods), P.O. Box 1427, 310 So. Extension Road, Mesa, Ariz. 85201

Sherman Foods, Inc., 276 Jackson Ave., New York, N.Y. 10054

Specialty Foods Corp., 1523 Nineteenth, Denver, Colo. 80202

Spice Island Specialty Brands, Inc. (Marie's refrigerated dressings), P.O. Box 2187, South San Francisco, Calif. 94080

Spreckels Sugar Co. (sugar), San Francisco, Calif. 94111

Standard Milling Co., Kansas City, Mo. 64109

Sterling Food Co. (soya, carob, flour mix), 5118 - 14th Avenue NW, Seattle, Wash. 98107

Sugar Lo (Parv-a-Zert, frozen desserts), 2001 Bacharach Blvd., Atlantic City, N. J. 08401. Attn: Alan E. Kligerman

Sugar Foods Corp. (Sweet'n Natural fruit sugar), P.O. Box 55086, Sherman Oaks, Calif. 91402 OR P.O. Box 410, Brooklyn, N. Y. 11202

Superose Sweetener (G. H. Whitlock Process Co.), P.O. Box 259, Springfield, Ill. 62705

Syntex Laboratories, Inc., Nutritional Products Division, 3401 Hillview Drive., Palo Alto, Calif. 94304

Tillie Lewis (low calorie specialties), Drawer J, Stockton, Calif. 95201

Tropicana Products, Inc. (pure orange juice), P.O. Box 338, Bradenton, Fla. 33506

Van Brode Milling Co., Clinton, Mass 01510

Vital Foods Distributors, 314 Second Ave., South, Seattle, Wash. 98104

U.S. Government:

- Department of Agriculture, Science & Education Administration, Consumer & Food Economic Institute, Hyattsville, Md. 20782
- Department of Agriculture, Research Service, Independence Ave. 12th & 14th Streets SW, Washington, D.C. 20251
- Department of Health & Welfare, Food & Drug Administration, Consumer Communications Staff, 5600 Fisher's Lane, HFJ, Rockville, Md. 20857

Worthington Foods, Inc. (Soyamel), 900 Proprietors Road, Worthington, Ohio 43085

York Barbell Company, York, Penn. 17405

Note to our readers: If you know of any edible products, especially for people with food allergies of which we may be unaware, we would very much appreciate hearing about it. Please write and let us know what you think of the product and give us their address. Thank you.

B.L.

INDEX

The number in parenthesis after each recipe title refers to the part of book in which that particular recipe will be found.

S

ABOUT THE AUTHOR

BILLIE LITTLE, a former East Coast newspaperwoman, is now a resident of California, where she occupies herself with writing cookbooks. She comes by her interest in food allergies naturally. Her mother had food allergies, her son is allergic, and so, in fact, is she. She is also the author of *Recipes for Diabetics*.

"I'd like to thank each and every one of you for signing my petition, and for your support on this drive," Mollie called out.

The group surged closer to Mollie, clapping and whistling their approval. "That brings me to my big announcement," she continued, when the applause had settled down. "It's about our friend, Ken Tilson." She gestured grandly toward Ken, who looked surprised.

"Some of you may not know this but, before his accident, Ken was a great tennis player. And I'm sure he still is. Just because you're in a wheelchair doesn't mean you're not an athlete anymore. And to prove it, Ken will be representing Vista High in the National Foundation of Wheelchair Tennis Tournament, which takes place two weeks from today!"

This time the roar was deafening. As Mollie led the cheering, well-wishers swarmed around Ken, clapping him on the back and shaking his hand. Mollie looked over at him proudly to catch his reaction.

Ken was sitting absolutely stock-still. The smile had completely faded from his face and he stared in disbelief at Mollie. His jaw was taut with fury and she thought the anger in his eyes would burn a hole through her.

FAWCETT GIRLS ONLY BOOKS

SISTERS

THREE'S A CROWD #1

TOO LATE FOR LOVE #2

THE KISS #3

SECRETS AT SEVENTEEN #4

ALWAYS A PAIR #5

ON THIN ICE #6

STAR QUALITY #7

MAKING WAVES #8

TOO MANY COOKS #9

OUT OF THE WOODS #10

NEVER A DULL MOMENT #11

SISTERS

NEVER A DULL MOMENT

Jennifer Cole

FAWCETT GIRLS ONLY • NEW YORK

RLI: $\frac{\text{VL: Grades 5 + up}}{\text{IL: Grades 6 + up}}$

A Fawcett Girls Only Book
Published by Ballantine Books
 Published in the United States by Ballantine Books, a division of Random House, Inc., New York, and simultaneously in Canada by Random House of Canada Limited, Toronto.

Library of Congress Catalog Card Number: 86-91823

ISBN 0-449-13211-0

Manufactured in the United States of America

First Edition: May 1987

This is for Ken Tillotson

Chapter 1

"*Ugh! Monday morning,*" Mollie Lewis said grumpily as she shuffled into the kitchen and slumped down at the table across from her sister Cindy. She exhaled a large, heartfelt sigh and rested her chin in her hands.

Cindy flipped to the next page of *Surfer* maggazine and completely ignored her younger sister.

"What an awful day," Mollie moaned, this time a little louder.

"What are you talking about?" a voice chirped from behind her. "It's gorgeous outside."

Mollie looked up just as her oldest sister swept into the kitchen. Nicole threw open the curtain, letting in streams of sunlight that shone off her chestnut-brown hair.

"Look at that sky! There's not a cloud in it!"

Nicole gestured toward the window and smiled down at Mollie.

"I don't think Mollie is referring to the weather," Cindy commented, keeping her eyes focused on the magazine.

"Ah, je comprends," Nicole trilled in her best French accent. Nicole was absolutely obsessed with everything French and never missed an opportunity to throw in a comment in that language, much to the irritation of her sisters. "I understand."

Mollie tossed her curly blond hair over her shoulders and slumped farther down in her chair.

"Want some breakfast?" Nicole asked, patting Mollie on the shoulder. "Maybe some food would cheer you up."

"I can only have half a grapefruit," Mollie grumbled. "It's part of my new diet."

"What happened to the protein milkshakes?" Cindy asked as she took a large bite out of her cinnamon toast.

"Or the eat-all-the-bananas-you-want diet?" Nicole added.

"I quit those weeks ago," Mollie said, hungrily eyeing Cindy's toast. "Now it's just grapefruit and cottage cheese."

At fourteen, Mollie still had a little baby fat and she just knew that if she didn't watch out it would blossom into full-fledged flab.

"Cottage cheese for breakfast sounds totally awful," Cindy said, wrinkling her tanned nose.

Nicole shook her head and chastened, "I don't see why you diet anyway, Mollie. You've got a cute figure."

"You're a model. How could *you* understand?" Mollie rolled her big blue eyes at her sister. "I mean, you've never had to worry about fat a day in your life. It's just not fair."

Nicole started to protest, but Mollie continued listing her grievances, ticking them off on her fingers as she said them. "You guys got all the good traits in the family. Cindy is the athlete. The best surfer in Santa Barbara, the fastest swimmer, the strongest arm wrestler—"

Cindy flexed her bicep jokingly while Nicole laughed.

"And Nicole is Miss Perfect!" Mollie shouted above their snickering. "Perfect figure, perfect grades, perfect leader— "

"And you are perfectly nuts!" Nicole reached over and ruffled her hair.

"You see?" Mollie protested. "No one ever takes me seriously."

"Look who got up on the wrong side of the bed," Cindy muttered sarcastically.

"That's not true," Mollie retorted. Then she leaned forward and declared, "I just want to be good at something like you guys, have people take me seriously."

"Well, have you thought about what you could do to achieve that?" Nicole said, humoring her sister.

"Um, well, yeah. Kind of. I'd like to do something that helps people. Like Norma Rae."

"Who's Norma Rae?" Cindy asked. "Is she new in your class?"

"Of course not, silly." Mollie's blue eyes flashed as she explained, "Norma Rae was a courageous labor leader in the South. I saw her on TV last night at Sarah's house on a program we had to watch for civics class."

"That's a movie, Mollie," Cindy said impatiently, taking a big gulp of milk. "It's just make-believe."

"Well, she seemed real, and her cause was real," Mollie said defiantly. "She was someone who made a difference in people's lives."

"But, Mollie," Nicole said, putting on her Big Sister voice, "you do make a difference, a big difference, in all of our lives."

"I do?" Mollie asked, perking up.

"Sure," Cindy agreed, patting her warmly on the back. "Why if it weren't for you, things could get pretty dull around here."

"Really?" Mollie asked, a little more cautiously. There was something about the smile on Cindy's face that made her doubtful.

"Really!" Cindy grinned wickedly. "Remember when Grant and I had that misunderstanding? We probably would have made up with no problem if you hadn't locked us in that tool cabinet. We almost killed each other." She smiled sweetly at Mollie. "Instead, we decided to kill you."

"Cindy's absolutely right," Nicole chimed in.

"Remember when you nearly ended my modeling career before it began? You knocked over a whole table of props and almost got me fired!"

"Now that you mention it, shrimp," Cindy concluded, "our lives would be very boring if you weren't around."

"That's not what I meant." Mollie folded her arms and slumped down in her chair. In the Lewis household it always seemed as if it was two against one—with her being the one. And just because she was the youngest.

"You two think you're so smart!" Mollie burst out suddenly. "Well, there are more important things in life than surfing or posing for fashion magazines!" She hopped up and shoved her chair under the table. "I don't need to stick around and have you two make fun of me!"

With that, Mollie marched into the hall with her head held high. Flinging open the front door, she shouted, "Maybe I'll see you at school, and maybe I won't!"

After the door shut, Cindy and Nicole stared at each other in amazement. Then they burst out laughing.

"What do you want to bet," Cindy said, "that she'll come home from school with an application for the Peace Corps?"

Nicole laughed in agreement.

"I mean, it's just another phase she's going through," Cindy continued.

"Oui," Nicole concurred. "One day she's run-

ning a home for stray dogs and the next she's decided to be an actress!"

That afternoon, Mollie stood on the steps in front of the school library, soaking up the sun and letting the warm breeze ruffle her hair. She smiled and gave the book tucked beneath her arm a reassuring pat.

"Remarkable Women," she murmured, saying the title aloud. *"Five Who Changed History."*

Mrs. Phelps, the librarian, had helped her find it for the civics-class paper she had to write. Mollie had spent the last hour completely absorbed in the life of Jane Addams, the founder of Hull House, and now she was busy imagining herself as the famous heroine, helping the destitute, fighting injustice with unflappable courage. She felt so inspired, Mollie just knew she had the fire and spirit to accomplish something as important as Jane Addams had.

She squinted into the afternoon sunlight and glanced around the Vista High campus. Students milled around the grassy hills in front of the school, some reading, some playing with Frisbees, others just chatting in groups.

In the distance she could see a typical Santa Barbara neighborhood—low white adobe houses with red-tiled roofs sat on either side of the wide tree-lined streets. It was beautiful.

Mollie's spirits immediately plummeted back to earth. How could she ever change the world when everything looked so perfect? "I'm a crusader without a cause," she muttered as she trudged up the short hill separating the library from the main part of the school.

Halfway up the slope, Mollie noticed a young man in a wheelchair, laboring up the hill ahead of her.

"Here, I'll give you a hand," she called out. In two quick strides she was behind him. She placed her hands behind his shoulders and gave the chair a tremendous shove.

"Hey!" the boy shouted as he lurched forward in his seat. "What are you doing?"

"Don't worry," Mollie yelled, "we'll be at the top in no time."

"Stop it!" he ordered fiercely. "Stop it right now!"

The ungrateful tone in his voice shocked Mollie and she quickly leaped back, letting go of his chair. Her movement was so abrupt that he was knocked off balance and nearly fell out.

"I'm sorry," Mollie apologized, not sure what she'd done wrong. "I thought you needed help. I mean, it looked like you were having trouble."

"I was going slowly," the boy explained, his voice tight with anger, "because I had a Coke in my lap and I didn't want to spill it!" He pointed at his lap. The cup had fallen over and soaked his jeans.

"Oh, no! I'm really sorry," Mollie stammered,

feeling like a complete and total idiot. "But I was only trying to—"

"When I need help," the boy snapped, "I'll ask for it." He batted away bits of ice from his pants onto the grass.

Mollie just wanted to sink into the ground. Tears stung her eyes and she stood there helplessly, unable to think of anything to say.

Then the boy looked up into her face and his frown melted. Mollie bit her lip and stared into his light-brown eyes.

With a sudden start she realized that he was very handsome, with his tanned, rugged face and curly dark hair.

"I know you were just trying to help," he said gently, "and I appreciate the consideration." Mollie looked up greatfully and he flashed her a sparkling smile. "But next time, look before you leap, okay?"

"I'll remember." She nodded. "But what about your jeans?"

He looked down at his lap and shrugged his shoulders. "It's a warm afternoon. They'll dry. Besides"—he grinned shyly—"it's not the first time I've been soaked by a good samaritan."

The boy flipped his chair around, with two expert pushes, and sped off toward the gymnasium.

"See you later," he shouted over his shoulder. Mollie waved in reply, even though she knew he couldn't see her.

She shook her head in frustration and moved

toward the bike racks. Nicole and Cindy were right. Every time Mollie tried to help out, she only made matters worse.

She stared out vacantly into space, idly rummaging through her purse until her fingers found the Snickers bar she'd been carrying around for the past week. She tore off the wrapper and took a big bite.

"Oh, no," she moaned, remembering that earlier that week she'd vowed not to eat another candy bar until she lost ten pounds. "That's just great," Mollie complained bitterly. "I'm a failure at everything. Even dieting."

She looked down at the half-eaten candy bar, debating whether to throw it away or finish it. She casually glanced around to see if anyone was watching.

Then, with one tremendous bite, she finished it off and dropped the wrapper in the trash can.

Chapter 2

"Lewis!" Coach Lawford barked that Monday afternoon. "You're late!"

Cindy Lewis scampered across the concrete deck of the pool, tucking her unruly blond hair under her swim cap.

"I'm really sorry, Coach," she apologized, adjusting her goggles with a quick snap. The other girls on the Vista High swim team were already in their lanes, waiting for the whistle that began the workout.

"Lane one," Coach Lawford said tersely, "four hundred yards, choice, in six. Lead off!" He jerked his thumb at the lane and rasped, "Go!"

Cindy went. Her coach was obviously in no mood for excuses from his star freestyler. She dove off the side over the heads of the others and pulled away down the lane.

By the end of the first lap, Cindy could feel herself calming down. The buoyant, slightly cool water refreshed her, and she luxuriated into the steady stretch and pull of her stroke.

Then she felt a gentle tap on her left foot. Involuntarily she dug in more deeply with her arms and the sudden surge pulled her away from her pursuer. But she was absolutely stunned by what had happened.

In the etiquette of swimming, a tap on the foot means, "Move over, I want to pass you." No big deal in itself—but no one on the swim team could keep up with the pace Cindy set naturally. That's why she always led off in her lane.

So who was hot on her heels? Cindy decided she must have been daydreaming and let her pace slacken off. That was one of the drawbacks to being the best swimmer on the team. There was no one to challenge you, to push you harder and farther. That was too bad, as far as Cindy was concerned. There was nothing she liked better than a challenge.

But Cindy usually won, no matter what the sport. Her easy athleticism gave her a confidence that was pretty unshakable.

As she flipped into her turn, she realized there was another swimmer only a few feet behind her. They almost collided as Cindy pushed off the wall. She hadn't expected anyone to be so close. Before she could recapture her rhythm, the tap came again—this time definite and insistent.

Totally confused, Cindy edged to the right and a flurry of hard-pumping legs and arms rushed by her with a *swoosh!* Cindy peered through the gurgling bubbles trying to identify her teammate. All she could see was a dark purple tank suit, rapidly moving out of sight ahead of her.

This is stupid, Cindy thought. What's she going to do, sprint the last one-fifty? She decided to teach the upstart, whoever she was, a lesson. Setting her jaw grimly, she set out to overtake the swimmer.

But to her total disbelief, she found she couldn't catch her. Cindy was practically going all out, yet the other girl steadily and methodically kept an easy length between them.

"This is only a warm-up," Cindy muttered to herself. "If she wants to exhaust herself before the real workout begins, that's fine with me." With that thought, she settled back into a more comfortable pace. But she couldn't control the rising sense of unease she felt in her stomach.

When she touched the wall to end the swim, she flipped back her goggles to get a better look at the swimmer. Cindy looked up to see her coach and the girl in the purple suit deep in conversation on the deck. She took note of the girl's unusually broad shoulders and muscled legs and shook her head in dismay. The girl radiated a sense of power and strength that was almost overwhelming.

"Looks like you've finally got some competition, Lewis," a voice murmured beside her. Cindy looked over to see Maureen Kilmurray grinning at her, obviously delighted by the new turn of events. Maureen particularly resented always playing second fiddle to Cindy on the team.

"Oh, I don't know," Cindy replied evenly. "Looks are deceiving, you know."

"Right," Maureen countered. "That's why you just finished eating her wake for four hundred yards. She giggled and Cindy felt her ears start to burn.

"That was just a warm-up," she shot back defensively. "Competition's another thing altogether." She hoped she sounded more sure of herself than she felt.

The coach turned and whistled them all to attention, mercifully cutting off the conversation. He grinned broadly and said, "I want to introduce the newest member of the Vista High Girls' Swim Team—Liz Wright. She comes to us from the Arden Hills Swim Club in Sacramento, so you can guess how glad we are to have her with us."

Cindy's ears perked up at the mention of Arden Hills, while her stomach sank. The club was world-famous. Mark Spitz, Debbie Meyer, and other Olympic champions had all trained there. Liz Wright was obviously no run-of-the-mill swimmer.

At her introduction, Liz smiled briefly at the other team members and quickly slipped back into the water in Cindy's lane. Cindy waded over to her side and stuck out her hand.

"Hi!" she said brightly. "Cindy Lewis." Liz looked up from tightening her goggles and stared at Cindy cautiously. Then she reached out and shook her hand firmly.

"Hello."

There was a long silence. Cindy shifted her weight uneasily in the water, then finally said, "Well, uh, welcome to the team."

"Thanks," Liz acknowledged before turning to listen to Coach Lawford deliver the instructions for the next section of practice.

Cindy listened with half an ear, still stung by the cold reception of her friendly gesture. She fixed her goggles firmly in place and prepared to lead off the next series. She crouched down, ready to push off the wall when the large timer got to zero.

"Lewis," Coach Lawford suddenly shouted. "Let Wright lead off. She'll set the pace."

Cindy stood up and gaped at him in astonishment. Liz simply shrugged and pushed off from the wall into the lane. Cindy started to protest, but Coach Lawford had already turned his attention elsewhere. She slammed her hand angrily against the side of the pool and followed her new rival into the deep end.

Suddenly a spasm ripped into her calf and she pulled up in agony. A cramp! Cindy couldn't believe it. She never got cramps. This afternoon was turning into a nightmare. She dipped under the lane dividers and dog-paddled over to the ladder.

"What's the matter?" Coach Lawford asked gruffly, his eyes betraying his concern.

"Oh, it's nothing," Cindy sputtered. "Just a stupid cramp." She pummeled the knotted muscle with her fist in frustration, then yelped with pain.

"I think you're pushing too hard," the coach said thoughtfully. "Go over to the diving pool and try to work it out." Then, as an afterthought, he added, "Maybe you should ease off on the surfing a little, okay?"

Cindy nodded and limped slowly over to the other pool. She gingerly sat down on its edge and lowered her legs into the still water. As she kneaded her aching calf, Cindy watched the swimmers, keeping an especially close eye on Liz Wright.

Her rival was the best swimmer she'd ever seen. She couldn't keep from marveling at Liz's capability in the water. She moved up and down the pool with a fluid efficiency that was very impressive. Unconsciously, Cindy started to imitate the angle of Liz's hands as they entered the water.

A voice broke into her thoughts. "I don't think that's your problem."

Cindy jerked back at the interruption. On the other side of the diving pool a handsome, dark-haired boy was smiling at her. Only his head and shoulders were exposed as he leaned his head back against the side of the pool. His outstretched arms, looped over the deck, had the smoothly defined muscles of an athlete.

"What?" Cindy mumbled, still a little confused.

"Your stroke entry. That's not your problem," he repeated patiently.

"What makes you think I have a problem?" she retorted.

"Well, I saw you trying to keep up with that fish out there," he said with a grin. "And I noticed that—"

"Wait a minute," she cut in abruptly. "Who asked you, anyway?" She pulled herself out of the water as quickly as her stiff leg would allow and glared at him across the pool. "I don't need any help, thank you, and when I do, I'll ask my coach for it!"

Cindy spun on her heels and stomped off across the concrete toward the locker room. She could hardly see straight, she was so angry. First, she'd been late for practice, very unusual for her. Then she'd been bumped from lead position on the squad by this newcomer. Then she'd gotten a cramp, and to top it off, some boy she'd never seen before had started giving her advice about how to swim. It was too incredible!

Who was he, anyhow? She'd never seen him before this afternoon, and she knew most of the guys on the boy's team really well. Cindy stopped at the door to the girl's dressing room and was just about to take another look at her critic when a loud whistle sounded from the main pool.

She looked over to see Liz Wright surging lengths ahead of the others down the first lane of the pool. Cindy set her jaw firmly and marched toward the showers.

"No question, Lewis," she muttered under her breath, "you've got your work cut out for you."

After practice, Cindy biked over to Pete's Pizzeria. Her gang usually hung out there when they weren't at the beach surfing.

"Hey, Cindy," a familiar voice sang out as she stepped through the door. "Over here!"

Duffy Duncan was bouncing up and down in a booth, waving his gangly arms like a windmill. Seated across from him was her boyfriend, Grant MacPhearson.

"Paging Miss Cindy Lewis, fabulous star of beach and pool," Duffy announced, holding a jar of grated cheese like a microphone. "Paging Miss Cindy Lewis. Your presence is requested at table four."

By this time every head in the place had turned to stare at Cindy, and she stuck out her tongue at her redheaded friend. They'd been buddies since elementary school and never tired of teasing each other unmercifully.

"Make way for the gimp!" Duffy bellowed as Cindy limped gingerly over to their table. Grant threw a paper napkin at Duffy to shut him up.

"No fair kicking somebody when they're down," Cindy complained, wincing a little as she slid into the booth.

"Aside from that phony limp you've picked up,"

Duffy said, eyeing her critically, "I don't see a thing wrong with you."

"I guess you'd better forget about medical school, then," Cindy retorted. "I got wounded today in practice."

"You're not kidding, are you?" Grant's blue-green eyes suddenly registered real concern. "What happened?"

"Well, I received a minor shot to the leg," Cindy said, massaging her strained calf muscle, "and a major blow to the ego."

"Don't tell me," Duffy cracked. "Someone forgot to tell you that you were the best."

"No, you creep!" Cindy lunged across the table and swatted him on the shoulder. "And just for that lousy crack, you're going to have to give me a whole slice of your pizza."

She scooped up the largest slice before he could stop her. It was smothered in pepperoni and onions, and the melted cheese was so stringy that it dripped all across the table.

"Not fair!" Duffy bellowed.

"You deserve it," Grant said, laughing. Then he turned to Cindy and asked, "So what's up, Cin?"

"Well," she began, "there's a new girl on our swim team. And as far as I can tell, she's not just good—she's great."

"That's good for Vista High," Duffy piped up.

"And bad for Cindy," Grant finished.

"Oh, I know it sounds silly, but I'm a little

afraid that I'm going to lose my place with the team."

"Aw, I'm not worried about you," Grant said, ruffling her short-cropped hair affectionately. "I've never seen a challenge that you haven't met head-on and beaten." He winked at Duffy and made a wry face. "Myself included."

Cindy tried to smile at his joke, but that uneasy feeling she'd had at practice was starting to creep back.

"Lewis," Duffy warned her sternly. "Either you down that pizza now or I am going to repossess it—with interest."

He grabbed wildly for the slice on her plate, but Cindy was too fast for him. She shoved the piece into her mouth before he even got close to it.

Chapter 3

"*Mon Dieu! I'm late!*" Nicole gasped after checking her little gold wristwatch. "Madame Preston will have me guillotined!"

"That's ridiculous," her best friend Bitsy scoffed as she pushed her glasses up on her nose. "If you tell her we had to meet a yearbook deadline, I'm sure she'll understand."

"I wish I could be sure of that." Nicole hastily gathered up her books. It was the third time in as many weeks that she'd been late for the honors French seminar.

Wednesdays were always crazy. That morning her mother had said, "You're involved into too many activities. You haven't allowed a minute for yourself."

It was true. Between being yearbook editor and

senior-activities director and modeling occasionally on the weekends, she really had no time for anything else but studying. There was certainly no room in her life for romance. Ever since she'd broken up with Mark several months ago, she'd hardly gone out at all.

Nicole shoved the printer's galleys into a folder and then called over her shoulder to Bitsy, "I promise I'll look these over at home."

"You'd better," Bitsy said, waving a threatening fist.

Nicole raced down the hall and paused just long enough to catch her breath and smooth her powder-blue cashmere sweater. Then she swept quickly into the classroom.

"Je suis desolée d'être si tarde, Madame Preston," Nicole apologized to her teacher and the rest of the class. "It won't happen again."

Madame Preston accepted her prize student's apology without comment and gestured for Nicole to sit down. Nicole took her place at the conference table the honor class used for its seminars. She looped her purse around the back of her chair, opened her notepad, and looked up directly into the warmest brown eyes she had ever seen. They belonged to the handsome boy sitting across from her.

Nicole felt herself blush at the frank admiration of his gaze. When he realized she'd caught him staring, he dropped his gaze self-consciously and looked at his hands, a small smile flickering across his face.

"Attention, s'il vous plaît," Madame Preston said, bringing the class to order. "This quarter we have a new member in our class. *Mesdemoiselles, messieurs, je voudrais vous presenter Ken Tilson."*

The new boy grinned and waved affably to the rest of the class.

"Now," the teacher went on, "I think we should spend today discussing what each of you intends to do for your project this quarter."

Nicole snapped back to attention. This was the quarter the honor students were to work in teams on special projects that they would research and deliver to the class. Madame Preston called them *"petites thèses"*—mini-theses. Nicole wasn't sure what she wanted to work on, but it definitely was going to have something to do with French art.

Madame Preston went around the room, and the other students announced their partners and their projects. When she came to Ken, she asked him if he had any special interests in French culture.

"Les Impressionistes," he said without hesitation, then burst out in English. "I mean, you could say it's an obsession with me, When I saw that exhibition in L.A. earlier this year, I—"

"En français!" Madame Preston broke in.

"Oh, right, *pardon."* Ken grinned sheepishly. He continued in French, and Nicole was impressed by his fluency and also by how knowledgeable he was about art in general. As soon as the bell rang, she stood up and introduced herself.

"Ken? Hi, I'm Nicole Lewis."

Ken was still seated across the table, stuffing his notebooks into a worn knapsack with "Stanford Medical Center" stenciled across it. He looked up and said warmly, "Pleased to meet you."

"Listen," Nicole continued quickly, trying to ignore the pleasant sensation that had come over her when he'd looked into her eyes again. "What do you think of doing a project on the Impressionists together? When you mentioned having seen the exhibition in L.A. earlier this year—"

"Did you catch that, too?" Ken broke in, his face lighting up.

"Yes," Nicole gushed. "It was fabulous. I mean, it's one thing to look at reproductions in a book, but to see the actual canvases was just overwhelming!"

Ken nodded in hearty agreement. They chattered enthusiastically for a few minutes, comparing notes and their reactions to the various painters.

"So, what do you say?" Nicole asked finally, when they'd paused to take a breath.

"I say, *Bonjour,* partner," Ken replied, holding out his hand. Nicole shook it and their hands clung together for the briefest second longer than necessary. Nicole hastily let go and grabbed her puse, holding it tightly against her chest.

"Listen, we need to get right to work on this,"

she observed, putting on her most businesslike manner.

"Well, school's out now. Maybe we can go get a Coke somewhere and rough out an idea."

"That'd be fine. We can go to Pete's—" Nicole slapped her hand to her forehead suddenly. "No, that won't work, I'm cooking dinner tonight." She cocked her head and asked, "What about coming over to my house for dinner? I'm sure it'd be all right. I'm making a special Provençal dish that's got to simmer for a few hours. So we could sit and work at the kitchen table while I'm cooking."

"Sounds great to me," Ken agreed with a grin. "I'll call my folks from your house and tell them I won't be home till later. Do you need a ride?"

"That would be wonderful," Nicole replied gratefully, turning away for a second to pick up her books. "I hate to walk anywhere if I don't have to. . . ." The end of her sentence died in the air as her mouth fell open in surprise.

Ken was in a wheelchair. She hadn't noticed it because he'd been behind the table when she'd come into class.

Ken saw the stunned look on her face and for a second the merry twinkle in his eye disappeared.

"Don't worry, I've got a car," he said impassively. Then he patted his chair and, with a mischievous grin, cracked, "Besides, this is strictly a one-seater."

As quickly as it had arrived, the awkwardness between them evaporated. Ken spun back from the desk and wheeled easily over to the open door. Without slowing down, he deftly popped the front wheels of his chair off the ground in a wheelie and bounced over the jamb into the hallway.

"Suivez-moi, mademoiselle," Ken shouted, spinning off down the corridor. "Follow me."

Nicole, still dazed, grabbed her books and scrambled after him.

"Here we are," Ken announced, rolling up beside the sleek new Toyota Supra parked in the school lot. He unlocked the passenger door and motioned Nicole inside. "Hop in."

Nicole stood awkwardly for a second, then asked, "Do you need some help?"

Ken looked up at her curiously but didn't respond.

"I mean, your, uh, wheelchair, and . . ." Nicole stammered. "How are you going to—?"

"Watch."

He wheeled around to the driver's side, unlocked the door, and deftly shifted his body onto the seat, placing his legs under the steering wheel. Then he grabbed the wheelchair and with a quick snap collapsed it into a compact unit that fitted easily into the space behind the front seat.

"Very impressive," Nicole marveled, sliding onto the seat beside him. He clicked on the ignition and the engine came to life with a roar. Nicole fastened her seat belt and watched Ken. The steering wheel had levers that allowed him to drive without using his legs. He slipped the car into gear and they rolled smoothly out of the parking lot and onto the road.

"That's incredible," she said. "I mean it was hard enough for me to learn how to drive using the pedals. If I had to do it all with my hands, I think I'd give up."

"It's not so hard," Ken responded, raising his voice slightly to be heard over the motor. "Besides, it's amazing what you can learn to do when you haven't any other choice."

Nicole nodded, suddenly embarrassed. She turned to stare out the window, biting her lip and trying to think of something to say that didn't refer to his disability. She realized she was avoiding using the words *walk* or *legs.* It was like trying not to say "See you later" to a blind person.

"Listen," Ken said, interrupting her thoughts, "you'd better give me your address before we drive all the way to San Luis Obispo."

"Mon Dieu!" Nicole exclaimed, sitting up with a start. "We should have turned left way back there."

"No problem," Ken said, signaling to turn around. "It gives me a chance to see a little more of Santa Barbara."

Nicole flung up her hands at him in mock horror. "You mean you haven't taken the grand tour of our fair city yet?"

Ken grinned back at her, skillfully easing the car through traffic. "We've only been here a little over a week," he explained. "Most of my time has been spent getting settled in the new house, registering at school. You know, all that stuff."

"Well, Santa Barbara is a beautiful town," Nicole said. "You really should see it. There's tons of stuff to see and do here."

"Perhaps some day soon *mademoiselle* will give me a walking tour," Ken suggested, turning to face her with an impish grin. Nicole felt her little fears of saying the wrong thing slip away as she fell easily into her new role as tour guide.

"Avec plaisir, monsieur," Nicole replied graciously.

"No," Ken said, "the pleasure would be mine."

Chapter 4

That afternoon, as Cindy came through the front door, she tossed her books on the hall table and took a deep breath. The house was filled with the delicious aroma of onions and potatoes and savory meat.

"Lamb stew," she pronounced to no one in particular.

Sounds of laughter spilled from the kitchen and Cindy smiled. Nicole and her mother must be whipping up something good.

Laura Lewis ran a catering business called Movable Feast and was always treating the family to some new and delicious recipes. Nicole seemed to be the only one of the Lewis girls to have inherited their mother's culinary talent, although a few months back, they had all tried to chip in and run the business while their mother was in the hospital with appendicitis.

A tremendous pounding from upstairs suddenly caught Cindy's attention. The thumping was coming from the vicinity of Mollie's room, so Cindy skipped up the stairs to investigate.

"Hey, shrimp," Cindy yelled, poking her head around the doorsill. "Whatcha doin'?"

"Redecorating," Mollie announced from atop a red stepladder. She didn't even turn around to greet her sister but kept hammering pictures to the wall across from her bed.

"What's going on?" Cindy asked in amazement. Gone were the posters of Matt Dillon and Mel Gibson that had plastered the walls. In their place hung peculiar black-and-white photos of stern-looking women in old-fashioned clothes and bonnets and a large poster of a wizened little woman wearing a faded gray scarf.

"Who's the old lady?" Cindy asked with a bemused grin. "And who's that woman carrying a candle?"

Mollie stepped off the ladder, and standing solemnly between the two pictures, turned to face her sister.

"This is Mother Teresa of Calcutta," she answered calmly, pointing to the old woman. "She won the Nobel Peace prize, you know. And this is Florence Nightingale, the founder of modern nursing. She was known as 'the Lady with the Lamp.' "

"Thanks for the lecture, professor," Cindy said

sarcastically. Then she shrieked in horror. "What happened to you?"

Mollie's normally wild, curly blond hair was pulled back severely into a neat bun at the base of her neck. She was wearing a black cotton skirt and a simple white blouse buttoned all the way to the top.

"Nothing happened to me." She sniffed primly. "I just decided that if I want to be taken seriously, I had better look serious. When I was a child, I thought as a child," Mollie quoted gravely, "but then I put away childish things."

"Wow, this is worse than I thought," Cindy groaned. "You don't have to join a convent to change the world, you know."

"Yeah, but every great reformer has had to make tremendous personal sacrifices," Mollie shot back, "and anyway, that's not the point." She moved past Cindy into the hallway, then turned to fling a final retort over her shoulder. Before she could say anything more, she was hit with the delicious scents wafting up from the kitchen.

"Wow!" She sniffed the air. "Does that smell good!"

Cindy burst out laughing at how quickly Mollie had dropped her somber pose.

Mollie completely ignored her sister's laughter and asked, "Who's cooking—Mom or Nicole?"

"Does it matter?" Cindy answered. "Either way it'll be great. They might be cooking together," Cindy added. "I heard lots of laughing in the kitchen when I came in."

"I'm starved," Mollie said, feeling a sudden gnawing in her stomach. "I think I'll just drop in and see if they need a taste tester."

"No, you don't, shrimp," Cindy roared, racing her sister to the stairs. "Me first, I'm older."

"Well, I'm wiser," Mollie shot back, sliding down the banister.

Before Mollie could reach the bottom, her sister tackled her from behind and the two of them wrestled their way to the landing.

"Well, I used to think my daughters were growing up too fast," Mrs. Lewis observed wryly as she watched the girls wriggle and giggle hysterically on the carpet. "But it's clear that reports of your maturity have been greatly exaggerated."

"Mom, that's not fair!" Mollie protested, trying to look as serious and grown-up as possible. This was a little hard because Cindy was sitting on her stomach and Mollie could only squirm helplessly like a turtle on its back.

"Face it, squirt," Cindy whispered wickedly. "Your cover's blown."

Mollie stuck her tongue out in response.

"Well, I just thought you both might like to know," Laura Lewis went on, "that there's a very handsome boy in the kitchen with Nicole and me."

"What?" the two girls cried out simultaneously.

In a trice they were both standing eagerly in front of their mother, begging for details.

"Whoa, wait a minute," Laura Lewis protested in a loud whisper. "I can only say that his name is Ken and that he'd like to meet you." With that, she turned and disappeared through the swinging door into the kitchen.

"Oh, this is awful," Mollie moaned. "I look terrible." She hurriedly loosened the top button on her blouse and pulled apart the bun, letting her hair hang naturally once again.

"What was that all about having to dress seriously to be taken seriously?"

"That had nothing to do with boys," Mollie said, smoothing her skirt. "Besides, I can be serious tomorrow. Right now, I want to look my best."

"Come on, Mollie. It's just a guy," Cindy scoffed, leading the way to the kitchen. Just before she pushed the door open, Mollie grabbed her arm and stopped her, whispering hoarsely, "Wait a minute. We have to talk about how to go in."

Cindy looked at her as if she'd just crawled out from under a stone. "What do you mean, *how* to go in? We just *walk* in. You know, one foot in front of the other."

Mollie shook her head. "Oh, Cindy. Of course you wouldn't understand something important like making a grand entrance. I mean, Joan Collins would never just 'walk' into a room. Don't you want to make a first good impression?"

"I think that's the dumbest thing I ever heard."

"Cindy, please!"

Something in the urgent look in Mollie's eyes made Cindy soften. She looked down at her sister and shrugged.

"Okay. What do we do?"

Mollie leaped into action. "First, we get a good look at him." She knelt on her knees by the swinging door and slowly pushed it ajar. A slender crack of light came through, and Mollie pressed one eye close to the aperture.

"Shoot!" Mollie muttered in disgust. "I can't see anyone but Nicole and Mom."

"Let me look," Cindy demanded, squirming her head into position just above Mollie and trying to focus on the source of the male laughter from the kitchen.

"Be careful," Mollie cautioned. "Don't push us into the room."

Cindy was about to reply when a loud thump from down the hall made both girls turn with a start. Before they knew what was happening, they were trapped underneath the hundred pounds of their playful, bounding Newfoundland, Winston.

"Winnie!" Mollie squealed, losing her balance and stumbling against the kitchen door. "Not now!"

But it was too late. The door flew open and a confused bundle of dog and girls tumbled onto the kitchen floor in an inelegant sprawl. From their places on the ground, Mollie and Cindy looked up sheepishly into three upside-down faces, peering at them curiously.

"Cindy? Mollie?" Nicole began by way of introduction. The two girls scrambled quickly to their feet as Nicole went on, "I'd like you both to meet—"

"You!" they blurted out at the same time, staring open-mouthed.

"—Ken Tilson," Nicole finished, a little confused by their sudden outburst. "He's from—"

"The library!" Mollie yelped.

"The pool!" Cindy stammered.

"My French class," Nicole broke in firmly. She turned to Ken with a perplexed look. "Have you met already?"

Ken looked at Mollie and Cindy and broke into a wide grin.

"We've bumped into each other," he said. His good-natured laugh melted their embarrassment, and soon the three of them were giggling uncontrollably.

Later that evening the Lewis family and their new friend sat down to sample Nicole's latest creation.

"Well, what do you think?" Nicole asked anxiously, watching everyone savor their first mouthful of steaming lamb stew.

"C'est formidable," Ken announced to the table, a large blissful smile crossing his face. "This is terrific."

"Appears you've made another gastronomic triumph," Mr. Lewis observed, beaming proudly at his eldest daughter.

"Absolutely," Mrs. Lewis agreed. "I think we can use this recipe at the shop without any changes. It's fabulous, honey."

Their mouths too full to talk, Molly and Cindy burbled approvingly while tearing off hunks of French bread to dip into the spicy stew.

Exhaling with relief, Nicole ladled a small portion onto her own plate and sampled her concoction. Immediately Winston was at her side nudging her forearm.

"Winston, that's terrible," she scolded, shaking her spoon at the dog sternly. "Bad boy! No begging at the table." Under her breath, she whispered, "I'll give you some later, you sneak!"

With a wag of his tail, the dog lumbered away from the table and collapsed in a heap by the door.

"So, Ken," Richard Lewis inquired curiously, reaching for the tossed salad, "what brought you and your family to Santa Barbara?"

"My dad's on sabbatical from Stanford," Ken told him. "He's teaching a seminar this quarter at the Renaissance Institute here at UCSB."

"Your father's a professor, then?" Mr. Lewis asked.

"That's right." Ken nodded. "And since I've already been accepted at UCSB for the fall, it seemed to make sense for me to finish high school here rather than back in Menlo Park."

"But wasn't it hard to leave all your friends behind?" Mollie burst in. "I mean, right in the middle of your senior year and all?"

Ken shrugged noncommittally. "It wasn't so bad."

Mollie and Nicole exchanged questioning looks. Then Nicole said brightly, "How about coffee now, and then a little dessert later?"

"No dessert for me," Mr. Lewis groaned, patting his stomach. "That was great, Nicole, but I think I've eaten enough for one day. I think I'll just crawl into my easy chair and see how far I can get with the newspaper before I fall asleep."

"We'll have our coffee in the living room, Nicole. And if Mollie and Cindy will wash the dishes," Mrs. Lewis suggested pointedly, "then you and Ken can get right back to work on that French project."

The younger siblings obediently stacked the dishes into the sink and got to work. Nicole poured out two cups of coffee, and slipping saucers beneath them, swung through the kitchen door into the living room.

"Mollie," Nicole called back over her shoulder, "would you bring the cream? I forgot. Sorry."

As soon as Mollie left the room, Cindy turned to Ken and said, "Listen, about Monday . . ."

He looked up at her, not comprehending.

"You know, at the pool," Cindy went on clumsily. "I'm really sorry I was such a—"

"I'm the one who should apologize," Ken cut in quickly. "I had no business giving you advice." He smiled at her shyly. "Especially unsolicited advice. So we're even, okay?" He held out his hand to shake on it.

"You bet!" Cindy agreed, gripping his hand with relief.

"So, how's practice going?" he asked, leaning back in his chair.

"Okay." Cindy shrugged. "I'm a little nervous. We've got our first big meet with Westside day after tomorrow."

"Westside?"

"They're our archrivals. It's kind of a big deal, and a lot of people usually turn out."

"Hey, I'd like to go," Ken said, "and root for you with the rest of your fans."

"Why don't you go with me?" Mollie said, suddenly reappearing in the kitchen.

"Why don't we all go together?" Nicole suggested from over Mollie's shoulder. "But now, Monsieur Tilson, we've got to get to work on our project."

"Right, Mademoiselle Lewis," Ken replied, saluting. Then he turned to Cindy and Mollie asked in a whisper, "Is your sister always this strict?"

"You don't know the half of it!" Mollie whispered back. Nicole jokingly shook her fist at them as Cindy pulled a giggling Mollie out of the kitchen.

Chapter 5

On Friday, Cindy stared numbly out at the rapidly filling bleachers of the community pool. It was the first meet of the year between Vista High and Westside, but more important, Cindy's first real head-to-head race with Liz Wright.

"Brrr!" Cindy shook her shoulders in an attempt to ward off a sudden chill. The prospect of possibly losing to Liz didn't make her feel too great.

All week long during practice, whenever Cindy had tried to go all-out and blow Liz out of the water, her performance had actually gotten worse. It was as if she'd forgotten how to swim. Cindy realized that she'd never really thought about swimming before—she'd just gotten in and done it.

Now all she could think about was beating Liz. Unfortunately the only thing she'd been beating lately was the surface of the water. Every stroke seemed a struggle, every lap a battle. And always there was the specter of Liz, cruising swiftly and easily through the lanes and leaving Cindy floundering in her wake.

"Hey, Lewis!" Duffy's familiar yell mercifully interrupted her train of thought. Cindy looked up and saw her redheaded friend and Grant waving at her from the bleachers behind the bench. Her friends Anna and Carey were sitting beside them. Smiling gratefully at the sight of a few supporters, Cindy loped over to her pals.

"Feeling okay?" Grant said, his eyes betraying the concern beneath the casual remark. "It's all right to have some nerves, y'know."

Cindy nodded convincingly. "I'll be fine."

"That's right," Duffy added emphatically. "This isn't a league meet, it's just a warm-up. Nothing on the line, nothing to lose—"

"But my self-respect," Cindy interrupted sharply. The boys recoiled a little from the brusqueness of her reply.

"Are you sure you're all right?" Anna asked, placing a comforting hand on Cindy's shoulder.

"I'm sorry, guys," Cindy apologized. "I know you mean well and everything. But I can't help feeling that I'm just a prisoner being thrown to the lions." She grimaced and added, "Or lioness."

The loud report of the starter's pistol made

Cindy turn around and see which race they were on. "Listen, I've got to finish warming up. I'm in the two-hundred-meter freestyle and it's next. See you later, okay?"

Grant put his arm around her shoulder and gave her a warm hug. "Win, lose, or draw, you know we're behind you all the way. Just give it your best shot."

Cindy smiled weakly and turned back toward the pool. Liz Wright was already standing behind the starting blocks, shaking out her arms and legs and stretching those powerful muscles. Cindy turned away quickly. Just looking at her rival intimidated her. She had to keep her concentration focused on the race.

"Two-hundred freestyle!" a voice boomed over the PA. "Ladies, take your marks!"

As Cindy climbed onto the block in Lane 4, she looked out at the bleachers once again. There was no sign of her sisters or Ken. Involuntarily she breathed a sigh of relief.

Good, she thought to herself. *At least they won't have to watch me lose.* As she realized what she was thinking, Cindy shook her head angrily. What kind of attitude was that? She had never thought like that before. Usually she was very sure of winning.

A movement at the corner of eye made her glance at the block beside her, where Liz stood poised to take off. She looked over at Cindy and grinned.

"Have a good race," her rival said, throwing Cindy into complete turmoil. She hadn't expected the sportsmanlike gesture and found herself mumbling a reply.

Before she could recapture her concentration, the start brought them to their marks and a quick set, and the crack of the pistol sent her springing into the water.

Her clean, shallow dive brought her almost half the length of the pool before she took her first stroke. Then Cindy attacked the race with a fury. With each splash of her arms she felt her body surge forward through the water, and she realized she was swimming faster than ever before.

At the far end she flipped smoothly into her turn and, coming off the wall, discovered that she was easily a full length ahead of her nearest competitor, Maureen Kilmurray. Liz was back another half length. With a surge of adrenaline Cindy redoubled her efforts and stretched her lead at the halfway mark to two lengths. She was almost laughing her way through the water.

Just before the final turn a horrible realization came over her. She'd set too fast a pace for herself. Her arms felt like lead weights on her body. It took more and more effort to pull herself through the water. Now she was breathing heavily after every stroke, instead of alternating breaths, knowing full well that each extra breath cost her a fraction of a second.

Just hang on, Lewis! she urged herself grimly.

As she prepared to make her flip turn into the final lap, she glanced to the side quickly to see where the other racers were.

With a shock Cindy realized that Liz was right beside her. Her rival had steadily eaten away her lead, and now it would be a duel down to the final lap. Cindy threw herself into the turn and shoved off the wall with all the strength she had.

But it was too late. She didn't have anything left. Liz pulled steadily away from her, and Cindy helplessly watched as she fell farther behind. Her aching lungs felt as if they'd burst any second, and now the water, so supportive and forgiving only seconds ago, seemed like a solid obstacle through which she desperately had to claw her way.

Ahead of her Liz reached out and touched the wall, followed by Maureen Kilmurray and a girl from Westside in the far lane. Finally, Cindy slapped the wall, finishing a dismal fourth. She draped her exhausted arms over the lane floats and gasped for breath, numb with shock. Soon the shock turned to humiliation as the magnitude of her defeat sank in.

Up on the deck Liz was surrounded by the other swimmers, all slapping her on the back and congratulating her on what must have been a great time. Coach Lawford strode up, beaming at his new star and gesturing excitedly at his stop-watch. A cheer went up among the crowd swirling around Liz, and suddenly Cindy felt terribly alone.

"Miss?" a man's voice sounded from above her. She looked up into the eyes of the starter, Mr. Pinsky.

"Are you in the hundred-meter backstroke?" he asked.

Cindy shook her head slowly.

"Then please leave the pool. We've got to set up the next race."

Cindy nodded dully and pulled herself out of the water onto the deck. She couldn't bear to watch the celebration at the bench any longer. And the fact that her friends had watched it all only made things worse.

How could she look them in the face after this? She had to get out of there fast. Without looking right or left, Cindy grabbed her towel and ran through the swinging door into the girls' locker room.

She was thankful there was no one there. She leaned heavily against the lockers. Outside, the next race was announced, and the distant crack of the pistol signaled the new start. The cheers of the roaring crowd rang mockingly in her ears.

I can't go back out there! Cindy thought. It's too humiliating. She changed into her street clothes and slipped quietly out of the gym.

Chapter 6

"*I can't believe it!*" *Mollie fumed as she scooted* her chair under a table at Pete's Pizzeria. "How can they call it a community pool when the whole community can't even use it?"

The sisters' plan of taking Ken to Cindy's meet had completely fallen through. When they tried to get into the spectator section of the pool, Ken had discovered that it wasn't wheelchair-accessible. In fact, the only level way to the poolside was through the dressing rooms. But the boys' was locked up tight, and since the girls' was in use for the meet, they'd been told that it was off limits.

Nicole suggested that they wait for Cindy at Pete's. Then they discovered that because of the steps, the only way Ken could get into the restaurant was through the kitchen. Mollie and Nicole had gone with him down the back alley past the garbage-filled dumpster.

"There ought to be a law!" Mollie continued, banging her fist on the table. "I mean, somebody should do something!"

Ken watched her quietly, a glint of detached amusement in his eyes.

"Is it always this hard to do things?" Nicole asked him, as they scanned their menus.

"Not always," Ken replied. "Sometimes it's worse."

"What?" Mollie screeched indignantly. "That's just not fair!"

"You're telling me," Ken agreed with a thin laugh. "But I've generally found that if I want to do something badly enough or get somewhere badly enough, I find a way."

Their waitress arrived and waited patiently while they argued amiably over what to order. Finally they reached a decision.

"We'll have the Pete's Super Combo pizza," Nicole said, "with everything but anchovies on it. And I'll have a Diet Coke."

The waitress looked at Mollie and raised her eyebrow. "Same thing for me, thanks," Mollie said quickly.

"And what would your friend like to drink?" the woman asked, without looking directly at Ken.

Mollie's mouth fell open at the woman's rudeness. Nicole started to stammer a reply, but Ken spoke first.

"Their 'friend' would like an iced tea," Ken answered crisply, looking the waitress straight in the eye. "Go easy on the ice."

"Oh," the startled woman replied. "Right." Clearly flustered, she beat a hasty retreat toward the kitchen.

"It's things like that," Ken said after the waitress had gone, "that really get to me. A lot more than the few steps I can't climb."

"Why wouldn't she look at you?" Mollie demanded. Her initial astonishment was rapidly turning to outrage.

"It could be one of two things," Ken explained patiently. "Either she doesn't want to be accused of staring, so she ignores me completely, or she thinks that when I lost the use of my legs, my brain went, too." He crossed his eyes and grinned at them goofily. Mollie and Nicole giggled in spite of themselves.

"So you haven't always been in a wheelchair?" Nicole asked.

Ken shook his head. "No. Just a year and a half. It was the result of a car accident."

"Boy, you sure know how to work that chair," Mollie said with respect. "I mean after such a short time and all."

"I picked up most of it during the six months I spent in P.T."

"P.T.?" Mollie echoed, a perplexed look on her face.

"Physical therapy."

As Ken talked, Mollie rested her chin on her hand and stared at him adoringly. Nicole watched her hang on his every word and groaned inwardly. That "my hero!" look in her sister's eyes could only mean trouble. There was no telling to what lengths Mollie would go to impress him.

Nicole's musing was interrupted by the arrival of the waitress with their order. Just as she was setting the steaming pizza down between them, Duffy and Grant appeared at their table.

"Hey, hey, hey," Duffy chortled, ravenously eyeing the hot pizza. "Looks like we're just in time."

"Duffy Duncan, you get your own pizza!" Mollie ordered. "This is for me and Nicole—and our friend Ken Tilson." She gestured proudly toward Ken.

After Nicole had made the introductions, Grant pulled up some chairs from another table. Duffy looked at Ken intently for a moment. Finally, he asked, "Haven't we met before?"

"No," Ken replied, with a shake of his head. "I don't think so."

"Gee, you sure look familiar," the redhead insisted.

"I'm positive you couldn't have met," Mollie broke in authoritatively. "Ken just moved here. He's from Menlo Park."

She beamed over at Ken as if he were her own private discovery. "Hey, where's Cindy?" Nicole asked. "Didn't she come with you guys?"

"Actually," Grant confessed, "we were kind of hoping she'd be with you."

"She usually likes to come to Pete's to celebrate her victories," Nicole explained to Ken. "I wonder what happened."

"Well," Duffy said, looking a little uncomfortable, "she doesn't really have anything to celebrate."

"What do you mean?" Nicole asked. "Didn't she win?"

Duffy and Grant booth shook their heads.

"Oh, no. This is incredible. Cindy *always* wins!" Mollie declared.

"Not this time," Grant said ruefully. "There's a new girl on the squad and she's a real shark in the water."

"Liz Wright," Ken said.

Duffy turned to him in surprise. "How'd you know?"

"She's pretty well known up in the Bay area. Liz almost made All-State last year."

Grant whistled softly. "Looks like Cindy's got her work cut out for her."

"If I know Cindy," Nicole murmured, "I bet she's pretty upset. Being the best swimmer on the team is really important to her."

"Well, it was just the first meet," Grant said calmly. "She's got another against El Camino the end of next week. What do you want to bet Cindy will be back in winning form by then?"

"Can't keep a Lewis down for long, I always

say," Duffy mumbled, his mouth full of pizza. "Nothing like a little competition to get her fired up."

Nicole and Mollie laughed knowingly. They both knew how much Cindy liked a challenge. Then Mollie sobered.

"Well, I hope so." She pouted. "Otherwise she'll be a real pain to be around at home."

"Don't forget the party at the beach tomorrow," Grant reminded them. "That ought to cheer her up."

"Hey, I almost forgot about that," Mollie said.

"Ken, you should come!" Nicole insisted. "You'll meet a lot of new people."

"Yeah," Mollie chorused. "You *have* to come, Ken. It'll be great."

"And," Nicole added, "we can spend some of the time talking about our French project."

Ken hesitated for a moment.

"Please!" Mollie coaxed. "It'll be awful if you don't come."

"Looks like I don't have a choice," Ken said with a laugh.

"Great," Nicole said, digging for a pen in her purse. "I'll jot down the directions for you."

"Here's a napkin to write on," Mollie said, shoving one in front of her sister.

"Now, the food's already settled," Nicole spoke as she wrote. "But everyone is bringing something to drink." She looked up at him and smiled. "You should also bring a good sun screen."

"And a towel," Mollie added.

Ken shook his head in wonder at the sisters' efficiency.

"My friend," Grant said, smiling broadly at Ken, "you've just been hit by the Lewis Blitz!"

"No kidding," Ken responded good-naturedly. "I know when I've met my match!"

"Match! Hey, I've got it!" Duffy shouted, choking on a piece of pepperoni. His eyes watered and Grant and Nicole pounded him on the back.

When he finally stopped coughing, Duffy looked across the table at Ken and announced triumphantly, "*Sports Illustrated,* Newsmakers Section, maybe two years ago. Ken Tilson, fifteen years old, youngest player ever to win the Alta California Open Junior Tennis Tournament." Then he threw open his arms and asked smugly, "Am I right or what?"

Ken nodded but didn't say anything. He kept his eyes focused steadily on his plate.

"You were written up as the best junior tennis player since John McEnroe," Duffy crowed. "You didn't lose a single game, set, or match in the final."

"Boy, you've got some memory," Ken said, looking up at him.

"Naw." Duffy laughed. "It's just that I love tennis." Suddenly he furrowed his brow. "Everyone said you'd be a shoo-in for high school All-American. What happened?"

An embarrassed silence descended upon the

table. Nicole stared down at her hands. Ken looked at Duffy for a second and then, with one push of his hand, rolled his chair back from the table.

A long minute passed.

"Can I die now?" Duffy finally muttered. "A simple bullet to the head will do. Maybe I'll just choke on this foot in my mouth."

Ken stared at him straight-faced for a moment and then burst out laughing. Nicole and Mollie joined him. They had never seen Duffy look so flustered. The color of his face almost matched his red hair.

"Hey, Duffy, don't worry about it," Ken said. Then his face grew serious. "It's funny. I try to put tennis out of my mind completely. Because it's the one thing I still really miss." Then he shrugged. "Once a jock, always a jock, I guess."

No one said anything for a moment. Then Ken broke the silence. "Well, guys, I think I'd better get a move on. I've got a lot of catching up to do at Vista High."

Nicole nodded her understanding.

"Aw, do you have to go?" Mollie asked, plainly disappointed.

" 'Fraid so," Ken replied. He took out his wallet and quickly counted out some bills. "This should cover my share," he said, placing the money beside his plate. Ken nodded to Duffy and Grant. "Nice meeting you guys."

"I'll give you a hand," Mollie said, starting to get up from her place.

Ken motioned her to sit back down. "That's okay, Mollie. I know the way out." Then he turned to Nicole and said, *"A demain?"*

Nicole felt herself blush as she answered, "Yes, see you tomorrow."

Ken's face brightened into a broad smile, and with a quick wave he spun off through the restaurant and disappeared.

"Nice guy," Grant murmured.

"Yeah," Duffy agreed. "What a lousy break, huh?"

As Mollie recounted in detail the problems Ken had faced that afternoon, Grant and Duffy battled each other for the last piece of pizza.

That night Nicole was busy writing in her diary when a soft knock sounded on her door.

"It's me—Mollie," a voice whispered from the hall. "Can I talk to you for a second?"

"Entrez," Nicole called out. "The door's open."

Mollie stepped into the room and closed the door behind her. When she turned and looked at her sister, she gasped. "Nicole, you look like you just stepped out of a painting."

Nicole smiled at her sister's compliment. She was sitting at her writing desk in her white ruffled nightgown. She'd tied a lavender ribbon around her hair to keep it back from her face as she wrote. The ribbon matched the bows on the satin slippers that peeked out from beneath the hem of her nightgown.

"What's up, Mollie?" she asked, closing her diary carefully and balancing it on her lap.

"I've been working on this letter," Mollie said, holding up a few pages of binder paper in her hand, "and I wanted to see what you thought of it."

"Who's it to?" Nicole asked.

"The school board."

"What?" Nicole gaped at her youngest sister.

"It's about the lack of wheelchair access at school." She flopped down onto Nicole's bed. "Ever since we got home this afternoon, I've been thinking about Ken and how we had to miss Cindy's meet because there was no way for him to get into the pool area.

"I've been thinking about Ken, too."

"Well," Mollie continued, "then I realized there were lots of places at school that Ken or anyone in a wheelchair would have trouble reaching. Like the band room, the practice rooms, the student-activities room, stuff like that. I made a list to send along with my letter."

"Read me the letter," Nicole urged. She folded her hands in her lap and settled into her chair.

Sitting stiffly on the edge of the bed, Mollie cleared her throat and began to read.

"Dear sirs—" She paused and looked up at Nicole.

"So far, so good," Nicole said with a grin.

Mollie giggled and went on with her letter. With each word her voice grew stronger and more resolute until, finally, she came to the end. She set the letter on the bed beside her and looked back at her sister.

"Well? What do you think?"

Nicole approached Mollie with a huge smile on her face and threw her arms around her. "Oh, Mol, I think it's wonderful." Then she stepped back and stared at her sister in amazement. "I can't believe you wrote it!"

"Well, it wasn't all me," Mollie confessed. "I had a little help from Mom and the dictionary."

"Even so, it's great." Nicole looked at her sister proudly. "You did a terrific job."

"Mom said she'd help me type it and then I can mail it to the school board." Mollie twisted her hands. "I hope they take me seriously."

"They will," Nicole declared firmly. A sudden thought struck her and added, "You know, Mol, maybe a petition would help make your point, too. You could get all the kids at school to sign it."

"Oh, Nicole," Mollie cried. "That's a grand idea. I knew I could count on you."

"I could talk to the seniors and juniors, and Cindy'll handle the sophomores."

"But it would still be my project," Mollie interrupted, a worried look on her face.

"Of course," Nicole assured her, mussing Mollie's hair.

"I can draw it up tonight," Mollie stated. "And start passing it around tomorrow at the beach party."

She jumped up and moved toward the door.

"Mollie," Nicole called after her. Mollie turned in the doorway and looked back expectantly.

"Did you hear Cindy come in?"

Mollie nodded her head, then whispered, "A long time ago. She hardly spoke to anyone. She just went straight up to her room and shut the door."

"She's not still upset about today, is she?"

Mollie shrugged. "She told Mom she thought she was getting the flu."

"Oh." Nicole nodded thoughtfully. "Maybe that explains it."

"You know Cindy," Mollie said. "She'll be okay."

"You're right," Nicole said. "She'll be able to handle one loss."

"Well, g'night." Mollie slipped out of the room and gently closed the door behind her.

Alone once again, Nicole picked up her diary and reread her entry for that day. She closed the book and leaned back in her chair, a dreamy smile playing across her lips.

Chapter 7

"Mom?"

Cindy stood at the bottom of the stairs in her nightshirt and peered down the hall toward the kitchen. It was Saturday morning and the house seemed deserted. She shuffled into the kitchen and called again. "Dad? Anybody?"

Still in a sleepy haze, Cindy threw open the refrigerator door, grabbed the orange juice, and took a long swig right out of the carton. At the same time she squinted at the clock on the stove.

"What?" she yelped in disbelief. "One o'clock?" She couldn't remember the last time she'd slept that late. Usually she was the first one up, and now there wasn't a sign of anyone.

Cindy slumped into a kitchen chair and was immediately joined by Smokey. She held the cat up to her neck and nuzzled his fur.

"Why didn't I wake up?" she asked, shaking her head groggily. Then it hit her. The swim meet! What a total disaster! Last night she'd tossed and turned in bed, trying to figure out what had gone wrong. Suddenly she remembered what day it was and where she was supposed to be.

"The big cookout!" Cindy sprang out of her chair, sending Smokey skittering onto the floor. The startled cat watched her bang through the kitchen door and bound up the stairs to her room.

"I can't believe I almost forgot," Cindy muttered. She hurriedly threw on her faded blue tank suit and a pair of shorts, then slipped on a T-shirt and grabbed her tote bag.

The kitchen clock read 1:05 when Cindy dashed out the front door, strapped her surfboard to her bike, and flew off toward the beach in a spray of gravel.

Within a few minutes she'd reached the top of the hill overlooking the beach. She stopped, inhaled a deep breath of crisp ocean air, and drank in the view.

"Look at those waves!" She whistled. "Great day for surfing."

Cindy tossed off the T-shirt and gym shorts she'd pulled on over her tank suit and stuffed them into her tote bag. then she grabbed her board and headed down toward the beach.

Off to her right, Cindy could see the cookout grill already in place. Around it Anna and Carey lay on a blanket, working hard on their tans. She recognized some other friends, and the dainty figure of Nicole, prettily posed on a patchwork quilt. She was deep in discussion with Ken, who'd attached an umbrella to the back of his chair.

"Hey, everybody!" she yelled as she passed the gang on her way to the water. All heads turned her way, followed by waves and shouted greetings.

When Cindy neared the water, she dropped her tote bag on the sand, took out a tube of zinc oxide, and smeared some over her nose. One thing Cindy absolutely loathed was a sunburned, peeling nose, and she often had one in spite of her precautions. She picked up her board and charged for the ocean.

"Cindy!"

A tiny figure in a flowered bikini was leaping through the surf toward her, waving a clipboard over her head. Right behind Mollie was her friend Sarah, carrying an identical clipboard.

"Not now, shrimp," Cindy shouted. "I've got a wave to catch." With that, Cindy let out a war whoop and threw herself and her board headlong into the surf.

Mollie watched Cindy's lithe figure disappear beyond the breaking waves and paddle swiftly out toward the swells.

"Isn't that just like her?" she said, sniffling, to Sarah. "Here we've been out getting this important petition drive off to a great start, and all she can think of is flopping around in the water."

Mollie's plan for the afternoon had been simple. She and Sarah would stroll up and down the beach, collecting signatures for the petition. Of course, if they happened to run into some good-looking boys along the way, so much the better.

They had just spent the last twenty minutes talking to two cute guys from a neighboring high school. Unfortunately, in the excitement of talking, the girls had forgotten to get their signatures. But they'd collected ten before then, and Mollie was thrilled with her success.

"Have you told Ken about the petition?" Sarah asked.

"No," Mollie said, "but now that we've got some signatures, I will." She raced up the beach over to Ken and bounded across the coolers, spraying sand over every sunbather in the vicinity.

"Watch what you're doing, Mollie!" Anna shouted at her.

"Sorry, Anna," Mollie apologized. "But I have something really important to tell Ken!" She carefully placed her clipboard on the nearest cooler and promptly kicked some sand over Carey.

"Mollie!" she sputtered, leaping to her feet. "I'm going to strangle you!"

"I've got a better idea," Anna said, grinning wickedly. "Let's dump her in the water."

As Anna and Carey leaped up from their blanket, Mollie squealed and tried to bolt. Within seconds they caught her. Tom Patrick, another one of Cindy's friends, ran over to help. He grabbed her legs and Anna and Carey took an arm each. Together they worked their way toward the waiting ocean. Mollie tried to kick and scream in protest, but she was giggling too much to sound convincing. With great ceremony, they dropped the squealing, squirming body in the waves.

"Nicole, isn't it about time for a break?" Ken asked, flipping his sunglasses down on his nose. He glanced up at the broiling sun and adjusted his umbrella. "I can't think straight anymore."

"It must be the heat," Nicole observed.

"Yeah." Ken laughed. "It's frying my brain."

"It might also be the fact that it's now three o'clock. We've spent two hours trying to think of a brilliant idea for French class." Nicole gestured futilely to the little crumpled sheets of paper that surrounded them. "And have come up with nothing."

The sudden *thunk* of the volleyball landing nearby made the two of them look up. The ball rolled toward them and came to rest between the wheels of Ken's chair.

"Your serve, Ken," Duffy yelled from his position near the net. With a grin, Ken scooped up the ball and punched it back through the air to the waiting players. Then he and Nicole watched for a while as the game resumed.

Duffy's team was getting walloped because no one could block Tom Patrick. He was tall enough to jump higher than his opponents and smash the ball over their heads. After giving up five straight points, Duffy hastily called his team into a conference. There was some muffled mumbling and a lot of giggling from the huddle.

"C'mon, Duffy," Tom taunted cockily from the other side. "Why prolong the agony? You guys haven't got a chance."

Duffy stuck his wiry head up out of the huddle and snorted. "Hah! You are about to become a victim of DAB."

"DAB?" Tom hooted. "What's that?"

"The Duncan Anti–Ballistic Missile Defense System!"

He clapped his hands and his team scattered to their positions. As the serve arced high into the air, Duffy ran forward and lifted Anna onto his shoulders. Another player did the same with Carey, and now two eight-foot behemoths faced the stunned front line of the Patrick team.

When Tom's first smash was deflected out of bounds, his whole team got into the act. Pretty soon every guy had a girl on his shoulders, and the volleyball game was completely forgotten.

"I like your friends," Ken said, grinning at their antics. "They seem like nice people."

"They are." Nicole laughed. "Crazy but nice."

"I mean it," Ken said, leaning forward to look at her. "I was just thinking that I've been here such a short time and already I've made so many new friends. It's great."

"I can imagine how hard it must be to change

schools so late in your senior year." Nicole paused for an instant. "You must really miss your friends."

Ken didn't say anything. He stared out at the ocean. A slight breeze ruffled his hair and threatened to blow all of their notes away.

"It was my decision," he said finally in a quiet voice. "I could have stayed in Menlo Park. It's just that—well, I feel like I've had two lives."

Nicole shook her head. "I don't get it."

"You know, pre-accident and post-accident." Ken's eyes darkened for a moment. "My old friends had a hard time adjusting to me being in a wheelchair."

Nicole murmured sympathetically and Ken looked at her. "No. That's not really true," he said. "It was me who had trouble. Once I came out of the hospital, I knew nothing could ever be the same. I wasn't the same. And I needed to find out who the new, real me was.

"But all my friends wanted to act like nothing had changed—like, somehow, nothing really important had happened. And they couldn't understand why I'd get so frustrated—with them, with myself, with everything."

There was a long silence as Ken examined a broken clamshell, turning it over and over in his hand.

"I guess," Nicole said slowly, "no one else can really understand how you feel—unless they've been there, too."

Ken looked at her closely, then nodded. Finally, he took a deep breath and said, "So, I decided I should just, well, start over." He smiled at Nicole. "Then when I'm more sure, I'll go back and renew old friendships. Everything takes time, I guess."

For a moment they sat there without speaking, just looking at each other. The waves pounded against the shoreline, lazily ticking off the moments. The breeze picked up, and the crumpled notes rustled against the sand. This time it was Nicole who looked away.

"Hey, what gives?" Duffy shouted, flopping down beside them in the sand. "It's a fabulous day, the waves are totally awesome, the company perfect, and you two look like you've just lost your best friend."

"What we have lost," Nicole retorted, "or are dangerously close to losing, is our minds."

"Two hours and not one good idea," Ken groaned and pointed at the wads of discarded ideas scattered around them on the blanket.

"Wait!" Duffy ordered, holding up one hand. "Put it in reverse. You lost me somewhere back there."

Nicole laughed and explained. "We're supposed to have a project for honor French and we can't think of a thing."

"Everything we toss around sounds so dry and boring," Ken complained.

"Yeah, that's the trouble." Duffy nodded in sage agreement. "Most of those things turn out that way. You guys should do something really different."

"Like what?" Nicole asked, a twinge of exasperation in her voice.

"Oh, I don't know. Like, have a party." Then Duffy leaned Ken's way and rasped in a stage whisper, "You have yet to experience a famous Lewis party."

"C'mon, Duffy, be serious!" Nicole frowned.

"Hey, wait a minute!" Ken said, snapping his fingers. "I think Duffy may have hit on something."

"What?" Duffy joked with a wry face. "Throw a big party and maybe your teacher won't notice that you didn't actually do a project."

"No." Ken laughed. "We could have a costume party."

Nicole looked at him uncertainly, a little confused. "What would that have to do with the French Impressionists?"

"It's simple," Ken explained. "Everyone would have to come as a famous artist from the time."

"That's mostly men, though," Nicole pointed out. "Aside from Mary Cassatt and Berthe Morisot, who have we got? Most of the members of our class are girls."

"You're right." Ken nodded. "That's a problem," He thought for a moment, then said, "People could come as either an artist or a character from a famous Impressionist painting!"

With each word his voice grew more excited. "Aside from using a lot of their friends as subjects, the Impressionists, you remember, were also obsessed with recording everyday life, people in the street, how they worked, how they played—"

"So we could tie the two together," Nicole added, getting caught up in the plan. "Then we could re-create an evening at a Paris salon, with the artists and their paintings."

"Only, the paintings will have come to life," Ken continued. "We'll try to make the classroom look like the gallery where the Impressionists had their first exhibition, back in 1874."

"All the way down to the food that was served," Nicole said excitedly. "And you and I can act like guides, explaining the importance of each character to the class. Oh, Ken, this will be great!"

She leaped to her feet and started pacing on the sand. "We can even hand out invitations with Impressionists paintings on them."

"It would be *the* party of the year!" Duffy chimed in. Nicole and Ken stared at him incredulously. In their excitement they'd completely forgotten about him.

"No way, Duffy," Nicole ordered sternly. "This is strictly for our French class. Nobody else."

"Hey, wait a minute, don't I get to come?" Duffy protested. "I mean, after all, it was my idea."

Ken looked at Nicole and raised his eyebrow in a wordless question. After a moment she nodded reluctantly. "Okay, Duffy, you can come—but that's all. Remember, this party is for a grade. It's going to be hard enough trying to keep Cindy and Mollie out of it."

"Keep Cindy out of what?" Cindy demanded curiously as she and Grant jogged up, sticking their boards in the sand and grabbing their towels. Yellow zinc oxide was smeared all over their noses, and Grant had drawn two stripes across each cheek, like war paint.

Before Nicole could respond to her sister's question, Ken smoothly changed the subject. "Hey, Cindy," he said with a genial wave, "sorry I missed your meet yesterday."

Cindy groaned and made a sour face. "Believe me, you didn't miss a thing. Just the slow and painful demise of Cindy Lewis."

"Aw, come on," Grant said, snapping his towel at her playfully. "That's not true."

"It is, too," Cindy said. "It was awful. Don't remind me." She scrunched up her face and slowly crumpled forward onto the sand.

"It couldn't have been *that* bad!" Ken laughed.

"Yes, it was," Cindy said, raising herself up on one elbow. "Maybe worse."

"One off day can't spoil the show," Grant said, helping Cindy to her feet and slipping an arm around her waist. "By the next meet, she'll be back on top, where she belongs."

Cindy forced a thin smile and stepped back to shake the water out of her hair.

"Hey, Cin," Nicole said, changing the subject. "With the help of your pal Duffy, Ken and I have finally settled on a project for French class."

"It's pure genius," Ken added with a grin.

"But we have to keep it under our hats," Nicole warned, raising a delicate finger.

"Okay." Cindy put her hands on her hips. "Tell me about this brilliant, top-secret idea."

Nicole and Ken quickly explained the party idea to Cindy, keeping their voices low. Then Mollie joined them, and they had to repeat the idea all over again.

"Oh, Nicole!" Mollie squealed, "that sounds great! You've got to let Cindy and me come!"

Nicole started to refuse, but Ken broke in, saying, "You know, they could help out. Be French maids or something."

The pathetic sight of her younger sisters' pleading face was too much for Nicole. "Oh, all right," she said, sighing, "but just you two and Duffy. That's it!"

While Mollie was deliriously jumping up and down in the sand, Cindy held back a little.

"What's the matter?" Nicole asked.

Cindy pointed at Grant, who was standing off to one side rubbing his hair vigorously with a towel, and whispered, "Couldn't Grant come, too?"

"Yeah," Duffy coaxed. "Grant and I could be waiters. I mean, what's a Lewis party without the famous team of Duncan and McPhearson?"

"Mon Dieu," Nicole murmured, putting her hand to her head. "This party is getting too big for the classroom."

"Why don't you have it at our house?" Mollie piped up. "I'm sure Mom wouldn't mind."

"Not a bad idea," Nicole agreed, chewing her lip thoughtfully. "Then we could really decorate it like a Paris art salon. And I'd have better access to a kitchen for the cuisine."

Her planning was interrupted by a loud clanging noise. Kip Evans was standing beside the grill, banging a pan with a spatula.

"Come and get it," he announced, cupping his hands to his mouth like a megaphone. Kip gestured grandly at the barbecue grill covered with sizzling hot dogs and hamburgers. "Grab 'em while they're hot!"

In a flash Cindy was on her feet, racing Grant to the food. Duffy and Mollie scrambled behind them, leaving Ken and Nicole alone. Within seconds the grill was surrounded by a hungry crowd.

"Cindy," Mollie complained. "Leave some mustard for me!"

"Where do you want it?" Cindy teased, wiping some off her plastic knife and smearing it on Mollie's nose. "Here?"

Mollie's protests were drowned out in the laughter. Soon more mustard was being applied to faces and bodies than to hot dogs.

With an exasperated sigh, Nicole shook her head and turned to smile at Ken.

"I guess I should have warned you," she said. "When you agreed to work with me on this project, you didn't know I had two silent partners as well."

"Silent is not the word I'd use to describe your sisters," Ken observed.

"You're right," Nicole said. "In the Lewis family, nothing is ever silent. Or simple."

Mollie chose that moment to streak past them, screaming at the top of her lungs and spraying catsup at Tom Patrick.

"One thing's for certain," Ken said with a laugh, "there's never a dull moment."

Chapter 8

On Monday afternoon, Cindy stood in front of the entrance to the school pool, trying to force herself to go to swim practice. Friday's defeat was still fresh in her mind, and the idea of facing her coach and teammates was unbearable. She couldn't go in there.

She backed away slowly, and before she knew it, she found herself marching through the big glass doors of Vista High out into the afternoon sunshine. Each step away from school and swim practice made her feel more and more relieved, almost light-headed. She took a big, deep breath and hopped on her bicycle.

"Coach is going to kill me," she murmured to herself as she sped along the road toward the beach. "But I don't care!" The wind whipped through her short sun-bleached hair, and as Cindy crested the hill, her spirits soared.

The gleaming bay was creased with parallel lines of booming waves, endlessly curling into shore. And along each curling wave, tiny figures balanced on their boards across the foam, then cut away and paddled back out to where the breakers formed. Cindy grinned with exhilaration. Surf was definitely up today!

When she reached the beach, she pulled her bike through the sand toward the lifeguard station, looking for a glimpse of her pals. She spotted Grant out beyond the breakers, sitting easily on his familiar striped board, waiting for the right wave.

Then he flung himself down low, paddling furiously until his speed matched the swelling wave. At the just the right moment he hopped into a crouch, then stood up, his arms outstretched. With the spray lashing around him, Grant looked magnificent.

Cindy never tired of watching him surf. He was pure grace on a board. Cindy always appreciated a good athlete, she reminded herself. So why did she feel so resentful of Liz Wright?

"Hey, Cindy!" She turned around to see Duffy toss his surfboard on the sand and jog toward her.

"How's the water?" she asked, casually flipping her sunglasses to the top of her head.

"A little rough." Duffy bent to the side to knock

the water out of his ear and then looked at her quizzically. "Hey, aren't you supposed to be at swim practice?"

"I didn't feel like it." Cindy stretched her arms over her head to limber up.

"You didn't feel like it?" Duffy repeated. "Does that mean you're sick?"

"Duffy," Cindy huffed impatiently. "I really don't want to talk about it, okay?"

Duffy took a step back, surprised. Then he called over his shoulder, "Hey, Grant, Cindy's here! She decided to skip practice today."

Grant stuck his board into the sand next to Duffy's and came up to join them. "This wouldn't have anything to do with the meet Friday, would it?"

"Maybe it does and maybe it doesn't," Cindy muttered, avoiding his eyes and digging her feet into the sand.

"Why let one little setback get to you like this?"

"Who said I'm letting it get to me?" Cindy snapped back defensively.

"Skipping practice looks like a pretty clear sign to me."

"I can take a day off when I want to!" Cindy voice got louder and tighter as she spoke. "I mean, for the last year I have practically carried the whole team and I never missed practice once. I figure I'm allowed to once in a while."

"Hey, calm down," Grant said, putting his

arm around Cindy's shoulder. "If you're upset about that new girl, maybe we can talk about it."

"I *am* upset and I don't need a lecture!" Cindy shouted at him angrily. "Who do you think you are, my father?"

She could feel her eyes starting to burn, and she angrily flipped her sunglasses back onto her nose. "I just wanted to take the afternoon off and spend it with my friends, but obviously I've come to the wrong place!"

Before they could say another word, she turned and ran over the hot sand toward her bike. She could hear Grant calling her name, but she didn't turn around.

Who were they to tell her what she should or shouldn't do? They weren't her keepers!

Cindy slid into her sandals and hurled herself onto her bike, almost running over the Good Humor ice-cream man. Finally she was alone again, pedaling hard up the road away from the beach. She decided an order of nachos at Taco Rio's would calm her down.

"That's right," Mollie said, fluttering her eyelashes ever so slightly at the good-looking senior sitting in a booth at Taco Rio. "Just sign here on line 257."

After circling around him all afternoon, taking her petition to all the other tables, she'd finally mustered the nerve to approach him and ask for his support.

"Thanks, uh . . . Patrick," she said, studying his signature.

"Listen, I think it's a good cause," he replied with a supportive grin.

"I do, too," Mollie agreed, tucking her pencil behind her ear. When Patrick DeSantis offered her one of his nachos, she demurely declined, even though she was starving.

"I'm sending a letter to the school board, and if I get enough signatures on this petition, they won't be able to ignore it."

"That's smart," Patrick nodded, biting into a chip. "Good luck with it."

"Thanks, Pat!" Mollie was floating on air. Here she was, conferring with the senior-class vice-president—and he was taking her seriously.

As Mollie reluctantly turned to move on to the next table, she waved back at him brightly. Without even looking up, she launched into her little speech, and wondered wearily if this was the way politicians felt when they campaigned for public office.

"Hello, I'm Mollie Lewis, and I wonder if you'd read this petition on a very important issue and sign it. . . ." Just then she raised her eyes and found herself staring directly into her sister Cindy's face.

"Cindy, why didn't you stop me?" she shrieked.

"I wanted to see how long it would take for you to stop drooling over Patrick DeSantis," Cindy shot back.

Mollie stuck out her tongue. "Not so loud, please." She looked around nervously to see if Patrick had overheard her sister.

"Sorry." Cindy shrugged. She was still steaming over Duffy's and Grant's behavior at the beach.

"Hey," Mollie said, grabbing a nacho and a swig of Cindy's Coke. "Aren't you supposed to be at swim practice?"

"What's it to you?" Cindy challenged, snatching her Coke back out of her sister's hand.

"I just wondered, that's all," Mollie replied, a hurt look in her eyes. "You don't have to bite my head off."

"Well, if everyone would just mind their own business," Cindy snapped, scooting her chair back and standing up abruptly, "this world would be a much better place to live!"

With that Cindy stormed out of the restaurant, leaving a stunned Mollie in her wake.

Nicole took a large bite of her apple and lazily turned the next page of her magazine. She was lying on her bed, indulging in one of her favorite pastimes—leafing through the latest issue of *Bon Appétit.*

The front door slammed, and the sound of footsteps traveled up the stairs and ended with the slam of another door.

"Hello?" Nicole called out quickly. "Mom, is that you?"

She was answered by loud crashing sounds

that caused her to shriek and nearly drop her apple.

Then a steady humming noise began to emanate from Cindy's room, right next door. Nicole decided to investigate. She slipped down the hall and peeked cautiously around Cindy's door.

"*Incroyable!*" Nicole gasped. There was Cindy, vacuuming her rug. She had shoved most of her furniture to the side and was attacking the carpet like a person possessed.

"Cindy," Nicole called out. Then she realized her sister had her Walkman on and couldn't hear her. Nicole called her name, a little more loudly, then reached over and unplugged the vacuum cleaner.

"Hey, what'd you do that for?" Cindy asked sharply, looking over to the door.

"I wanted to get your attention," Nicole said.

"So you've got it," Cindy pulled her earphones down around her neck. "What do you want?"

"I wanted to find out if you were sick," Nicole teased, leaning against the door and taking a bite of her apple. "I mean, the Cindy Lewis that I know would never, *ever* clean her room in the middle of the day. In fact the Cindy Lewis I knew would generally be at the beach or swim prac– . . ."

Nicole's voice trailed off into the air. She cocked her head and stared cautiously at her sister. "Hey, why aren't you at practice?"

"Why is everyone so concerned about my swimming?" Cindy exploded. "Don't you have anything better to do than spy on me?'

"Who's spying? All I did was ask one simple question," Nicole shot back. "What's the matter with you, anyway?"

"There is absolutely *nothing* the matter with me!" Cindy shouted, as she angrily rewound the cord on the cleaner. "It's this family, and this house, and that whole, lousy school!"

She shouldered her way past Nicole and ran down the stairs, nearly tripping over Winston in the process. He thumped his tail and anxiously stared at the front door.

"Forget it, Winston," Cindy grumbled at him. "Not this time." The big dog's tail drooped and he slumped down pathetically against the wall.

Cindy threw open the front door and nearly collided with her mother, who was balancing two bags of groceries and fumbling for her keys.

Mrs. Lewis looked up and said cheerfully, "Hi, honey! How was swim practice?"

Cindy stared at her mother in disbelief, then raised her fists to the ceiling and screamed, *"Aarrgh!"*

Mrs. Lewis watched open-mouthed as her daughter ran down the front walk and disappeared around the corner. Then she turned and, noticing Nicole standing at the top of the stairs, asked, "What'd I say?"

Chapter 9

A few days later Nicole hurried home after her last class and strode straight upstairs. Outside Cindy's room she pressed her ear against the closed door until she was satisfied Cindy was there. Then she stepped down the hall to Mollie's room.

The steady *thunk-thunk* of a music tape throbbed from inside. Nicole rapped firmly on the door.

"What?" Mollie answered shortly.

Nicole opened the door and peered in.

Mollie's room looked as if it had been struck by a tornado. Clothes were strewn all across the floor and bed, and right in the middle of all the chaos was Mollie, lying on her stomach with her back arched, trying to touch one foot to her head. She was dressed in an electric-blue leotard with hot-pink tights. Around her waist was tied a pink-and-white striped scarf, which matched her headband. Smokey and Cinders were curled up at the foot of the bed watching wide-eyed as Mollie twisted herself into different contortions.

"It's not good to interrupt a person's workout," Mollie huffed. Then she rolled onto her back and attempted a few situps.

"Well, this is serious," Nicole replied, turning off the cassette player.

"How serious?" Mollie sat up and squinted at her older sister.

"It's Cindy." Nicole sat on the bed. "I'm really worried about her. I mean, she has hardly spoken a word to any of us since the swim meet."

"Yeah, I tried talking to her," Mollie mumbled, trying to touch her head to her knees. She flopped back down on the floor. "She was a big grump and told me to mind my own business."

"I thought she was just avoiding us," Nicole whispered. "But it's everybody. I met Grant at school, and he and Duffy haven't seen or talked to her all week."

"Where is she now?"

"In her room, but I have a feeling that she'll probably go out soon." Nicole bent over and looked her sister in the face. "That's where you come in."

"Me?" Mollie asked. "How?"

"I was wondering if you could sort of follow her

this afternoon. You know, make sure she's all right."

"You mean, spy on her?" Mollie gasped.

"That's a strong word for it," Nicole said quickly. "Just keep an eye on her. I'd do it myself, but I'm supposed to meet Bitsy in a little while. We're late on our yearbook deadline."

Before Nicole had even finished her sentence, Mollie was at her closet, throwing more clothes on the bed.

"What are you doing?" Nicole ducked and just missed getting hit with a pair of shorts.

"If I'm going to be a private eye, I need the right outfit. I wouldn't want her to recognize me." Mollie held up a sleeveless turtleneck dress and announced firmly, "Spies always wear black."

"In the middle of spring?' Nicole laughed. "You'd stick out like a sore thumb."

"You're right," Mollie started pacing back and forth, weighing her options. "I should wear sunglasses and one of your big straw hats."

"What for?"

"To disguise my hair. Hair is a dead giveaway."

"Where did you hear that?"

"I read it in *It's a Crime* magazine. It's a very informative periodical."

"I'll bet it is," Nicole said with a smirk.

"Do you think a trench coat is too much?" Mollie asked suddenly.

"I think *you* are too much!" Nicole burst out exasperatedly.

"Well, tailing someone is a subtle art—"

"Look, Mollie," Nicole cut in, "I just want you to keep an eye on her, not create an international incident. Besides, by the time you decide what to wear, she'll probably have left the house."

A door closed at the end of the hall and they stood still, listening. Ever so carefully, Mollie tiptoed to her own door and peeked out.

"Oh no!" she whispered. "She's leaving right now!"

"Then follow her!" Nicole urged.

"What about my disguise?"

"Forget it! Just go!" Nicole ran to Mollie's dresser and pulled out the first thing she could find. "Here, put these on." She handed her a pair of paisley pants. Then she grabbed a yellow T-shirt with big black polka dots off the chair and threw it at Mollie, yelling, "And this, too."

"Are you crazy? I can't wear that!" Mollie hissed. "It doesn't match!" She tossed the clothes onto the bed contemptuously.

Nicole let out an exasperated sigh, then snapped her fingers. "I've got it. Come on!" Without waiting for an answer, she pulled Mollie out of the room and down the stairs.

"What are you doing?" Mollie screeched, as Nicole flung open the hall closet and rifled through the coathangers.

"Here, wear this." She tossed Mr. Lewis's trench coat on over Mollie's leotard and tights, rolled up the sleeves, and cinched the belt tightly around her waist.

"Now, I'm going to be at Le Bistro with Bitsy. Do you know where that is?"

"Sure do, boss!" Mollie saluted. "I'll trail Cindy and report back there."

They heard the back door shut, and Nicole gestured for Mollie to follow. From her bedroom window, Nicole watched Cindy wheel her bike out of the garage and pedal off down the street.

About a minute later, Mollie appeared in the shadows, hunched over the handlebars of her bike. When she pulled into the light, Nicole gasped. The trench coat flapped out behind her revealing the bright-pink tights underneath. And she was wearing a very bizarre hat.

Mollie zigzagged up the street, scurrying stealthily from behind one parked car to the next, until she reached the corner. Then she slipped on a huge pair of mirrored sunglasses and turned right.

"Mon Dieu!" Nicole murmured, putting her head in her hands. "What have I done?"

Cindy focused her concentration on a little black rectangle drawn on the backboard. Then she flipped up a tennis ball, reared back, and let fly a ferocious serve that slammed against the wall with a resounding *thwack.*

After a week of depression, Cindy was starting to cheer up. When she'd first started escaping to the tennis courts on Monday, she'd hardly been able to hold the racket in her hand. She was all bottled up with frustration—angry at everybody trying to tell her what to do, and even madder at herself for letting something as stupid as losing a swim meet get her so upset.

"Take that!" she growled between her teeth, smashing the ball against the backboard. The *thwack* of her ball was answered by a loud *thunk* from the other side. She fired another serve and heard the echo again.

Someone's over there, she thought, listening to the steady pounding. And they're really pouring it on. She ambled over to the wall and peeked around to see who it was.

She was surprised to see Ken in his wheelchair, a bucket of tennis balls at his side, smashing serves against the backboard with rocketlike velocity. There was a dark vee on his T-shirt from perspiration, and with each swing his dark hair flung a spray of sweat into the air. Even from that distance Cindy could see his eyes flashing with intensity and concentration.

His frustration at being confined to a wheelchair was all too visible on his face. He lunged wildly at a rebounding ball, and Cindy thought for a moment that he was going to jerk himself out of his chair and fall.

"Look out!" she called involuntarily.

Ken froze at the sound of her voice. Looking up

at her, he seemed embarrassed at having been observed.

An awkward silence hung between them, and Cindy groped for something to break the stillness.

"Hi," she said, her voice sounding artificial to her ears. Ken nodded in greeting. "I was on the other side," she explained. "Thought maybe there was someone I could volley with."

"No," Ken replied. "Just me."

Cindy nodded and the awful silence was upon them once again.

"You play tennis a lot?" she finally asked.

"When I can," Ken responded. "I come here 'cause it's got the best backboard in town."

"It does," Cindy agreed. "It's great for pounding out frustration."

"Yeah," Ken said softly. "I think I know something about that."

Cindy nodded again but didn't say anything. Then she took a few practice swings with her racket.

"Want to volley?"

Ken hesitated a moment, and Cindy added with a grin, "It beats a backboard any day."

"Sure. Why not?" he said. They found an empty court, and Ken wheeled to a position a few feet behind the baseline. Cindy loped over to her side of the net and shouted, "Ready?"

"Fire away!"

Cindy looped an easy lob in Ken's direction and he snapped it briskly back.

"Better put a little meat on your swing," he joked. "I don't want to fall asleep out here."

"Remember, you asked for it," she shouted, firing off a firm shot that Ken had to wheel off to his left to reach. The angle was too sharp and the ball whizzed by him into the fence.

"If you back up as far as you can behind the baseline," Cindy advised, "you'll have an easier angle to come in on your returns."

"Good idea," he yelled back. Within a short time they were hitting the ball back and forth with ease and Ken began to grin with enjoyment. They chatted as they played, the *whack* of their rackets punctuating each sentence.

Then, out of the blue, Ken dropped a bombshell.

"You can beat her, you know." His comment caught Cindy completely off guard and his volley slipped by her racket easily.

"What?" she yelled, trotting to the fence to retrieve the ball. "Who?"

"Who do you think?" he retorted, grinning slyly. "Liz Wright, of course."

The cocky tone of his voice made her temper flare and she snapped, "I thought I told you once—when I need advice, I'll ask for it!" And with that, she blasted her hardest forehand smash straight at him.

No one she played with ever returned that shot. Not even Grant. Certainly none of the girls. So it was a startled Cindy who watched as Ken easily returned the ball to the opposite court, with a wicked topspin that made it curl wildly out of her reach.

"That's a mean temper you've got!" he drawled, a wide grin creasing his face.

"That's one mean return!" she answered. They both laughed, and Cindy prepared to serve again. Then she stopped and looked over at him curiously.

"How?" she demanded.

"How what?"

"How could I beat her?"

"It's no big mystery," he began, "just something I noticed that day in the pool when you wore yourself out trying to keep up with her."

Cindy bit her lip to stifle a rude response and waited for him to continue.

"You're kind of an emotional person, right?" he said, seriously.

Cindy burst out laughing. "I guess you could say that."

"Well, your emotion affects your performance," he explained. "It throws off the synchronization of your stroke. You actually get worse when you get angry."

Cindy knew he was right. That's certainly what had happened during the race with Liz.

"But I always thought emotion fired me up," she countered, "that it made me more competitive."

"Right," he agreed. "But you have to control it, and not let the emotion control you."

"Yeah, I always get so angry," she muttered

with irritation. "I can't see straight. Then I don't know what I'm doing."

"There's nothing wrong with being angry," Ken shouted, banging his racket against his chair. "There's plenty to be angry about, believe me. But if it just tenses you up, you become your own worst enemy!"

Cindy looked at him thoughtfully and waited for him to continue.

"You know how good you are, Cindy. You've always won in the past. I think that proves that it's your anger getting in your way." He looked up at her suddenly and grinned. "Getting awfully serious here, aren't I? Sorry about the lecture."

He started to serve up another volley but stopped. He raised his hand, shielding his eyes from the sun, and peered off to the right.

"What's the matter?" Cindy asked, following his gaze.

"I thought I saw something move over there in the bushes." Ken shrugged it off. "I guess it just was my imagination."

Cindy didn't answer. She looked over at the hedge bordering the tennis courts. The bush was rustling suspiciously.

On a hunch she tossed a ball in the air and fired it as hard as she could into the wiggling leaves.

"Ouch! That hurt!" a voice squealed from behind a clump of bushes.

"I thought so," Cindy muttered. Then she said

in a loud sarcastic voice, "Look, Ken, a talking hedge." She circled to the right and gestured for him to wheel to the left.

They peered around the hedge and caught sight of a ridiculous figure in a large coat, funny hat, and sunglasses crawling toward the nearest tree.

"Mollie!" Ken exclaimed. "What are you doing here?"

At the mention of her name, Mollie shrieked and sprang straight in the air. She started to run but stopped herself and spun around to face him.

"You recognized me?" she asked in a disappointed voice.

"Why wouldn't I?"

"Well, I told Nicole that a hat would be the best disguise—"

"Did Nicole put you up to this?" Cindy cut in.

"No!" Mollie spun around to face her sister. Then she stammered nervously. "Uh, I mean, yes . . . but up to what?"

"Sneaking around and spying on people."

"Well, it was for a very good reason," Mollie blurted out. "She's worried about you."

Cindy balanced her racket on her shoulder and rolled her eyes. "You see, Ken," she explained in her calmest voice, "this is what I have to put up with. Two spying sisters. I think it is only fair to warn you that this kind of thing can happen when you get involved with the Lewis family."

"I can stand it," Ken said, laughing.

"That's not fair!" Mollie pouted. "You're going to scare Ken."

"If that getup doesn't scare him," Cindy declared, gesturing disdainfully at Mollie's clothes, "I don't know what will!"

"What getup?" Mollie asked innocently.

Cindy pointed her racket at Mollie's head. Mollie raised a tentative hand up to feel. "Dad's fishing hat!" she gasped.

It was covered with little plastic fish and rubber worms. At the crown, standing straight up, was a little red-white-and-blue anchor. Mollie hadn't even looked at it—she'd just grabbed the first hat she could find in the garage.

"No wonder people've been staring at me."

"Dad's not going to be too happy when he sees what you've done to his favorite hat." Cindy was referring to the new additions of twigs and leaves and the big patch of dirt on the front of the brim.

"Maybe if I hurry home," Molly muttered, picking up the bike that she'd ditched behind a tree, "I can get there before Dad does and wash it out."

"You're not going anywhere on that bike." Ken pointed to her rear tire. "That flat looks serious."

Mollie looked down and moaned.

"Why don't I give you a ride?" Ken offered. "And we can put your bike in the back."

"Would you mind dropping me at a gas station?" she asked, her face brightening. "I'll get some air, and then go on to, uh, my next appointment."

"Appointment?" Ken asked, raising an eyebrow.

Mollie made sure Cindy wasn't listening and then whispered mysteriously, "I'm supposed to report to Nicole."

He still looked perplexed.

Mollie gestured with her thumb toward Cindy, gathering her tennis balls by the net. "You know, inform her of the suspect's whereabouts." Then Mollie pulled out a battered notepad and added, "I've got it all written down in here."

Ken opened his mouth to respond but just shook his head and wheeled off toward his car.

Chapter 10

Nicole drummed her perfectly manicured nails on the lace tablecloth at Le Bistro and stared out the window. Where was Mollie? She'd gone out to follow Cindy over two hours ago.

Across the table from her, Bitsy pointed emphatically to her yellow pad and said in a strong voice, "And I think the pictures should all be put in upside down, to really grab the reader's attention. Don't you agree?"

"Sure," Nicole mumbled affably, her eyes still fixed on the passersby outside. "That'd be fine."

"Nicole!" Bitsy said, slamming her notebook shut with a bang and folding her hands in front of her. "I think you should resign as editor-in-chief of our yearbook!"

"What?" Nicole stammered, jerking back to attention. "Why?"

"Because," Bitsy explained, "in the last five minutes, you have just agreed to nursery rhymes on every page, photographing the teachers in rabbit suits, and using pink and lime green as the colors for our cover."

"Quel horreur!" Nicole gasped, shaking her head ruefully. "I'm sorry, Bitsy. I just can't concentrate today."

"I'll say you can't." Bitsy sipped her café au lait and then looked sharply at Nicole over her cup. "What is it? School? Your family?" She wiggled her eyebrows suggestively. "A boy?"

Nicole stared down at the croissant on her plate. She'd hardly touched it. She murmured softly, "All of the above."

Bitsy set her cup down on the saucer with a clink and said in a motherly tone, "Tell Bitsy everything."

Nicole ran her hand through her silky brown hair and sighed. "Oh, it just feels like everything is happening at once." She ticked off the items on her fingers. "Our French party is less than a week away and we haven't even begun our paper on it. This yearbook is making me crazy. Cindy is sulking around at home, and Molly has gone totally berserk about her petition." Nicole heaved another sigh and stared back at her plate.

"And?" Bitsy asked, peering into Nicole's face.

"And what?" Nicole blinked up at her.

"The boy!" Bitsy burst out. "You've covered school and family. Now tell me about the boy."

"What about him?" Nicole shrugged, trying to look casual.

"Do I know him?" Bitsy asked, her eyes glinting with curiosity.

"I think you may have seen him," Nicole answered. She felt herself blushing.

"Let's not play Twenty Questions," Bitsy ordered in an exasperated tone. "Tell me his name."

Nicole wasn't sure she was ready to talk about Ken yet. She'd only just realized herself that she had a crush on him. Talking about it out loud made it seem a bigger deal than it was.

But Bitsy was not to be put off. "Okay," she persisted, "just give me the initials."

Nicole hesitated, trying to think of some way to change the subject. She was rescued by a loud car honk from the street outside the restaurant.

As Nicole and Bitsy turned and watched through the window, a bizarrely dressed figure on a bicycle wobbled to the side of the street, having narrowly avoided collision with a pedestrian.

"That almost looks like Mollie," Bitsy said dubiously, squinting out the window. "But she would never wear an outfit like that."

"It *is* Mollie," Nicole groaned, "and that outfit is her disguise."

"Why would she need a disguise?"

"I made the mistake of asking her to follow Cindy, and see what she was up to." Bitsy raised her eyebrows at her explanation and Nicole quickly added, "It's a long, long story. I never dreamed Mollie would take it so seriously."

"I don't think *seriously* is quite the right word," Bitsy observed dryly, as they watched Mollie lock the bike, pull her hat down over her forehead, and look to the right and then to the left. She scribbled something onto a pad of notebook paper and stuffed it into her pocket before stepping resolutely toward the entrance of Le Bistro.

"She's not coming in here, is she?" Bitsy exclaimed, looking positively horrified at the thought.

In answer to her question, Mollie made her entrance into the restaurant. Sliding her sunglasses down onto the tip of her nose, she peered mysteriously around the room until she spotted Nicole. Then she made a beeline for their table. Without even saying hello, Mollie flipped back the pages on her little lined notepad and began to read.

"The suspect was last seen playing tennis over on Manzanita Drive. However, due to a tactical error on the part of this operative, she spotted me, and my cover was blown."

People in the restaurant were staring at Mollie, and Nicole whispered urgently, "Mollie, please, sit down and speak English, not your crime-story lingo."

Without skipping a beat, Mollie flopped down into an empty chair and continued her report. "At first, I lost the subject—I mean, Cindy—but due to my keen powers of observation, I had noticed she was carrying a tennis racket and thereby deduced she must be going to play tennis."

"Way to go, Sherlock," Bitsy muttered sarcastically.

"So," Mollie continued, "I went to every tennis court in town until I finally caught up with her at the courts on Manzanita. She was playing with a Mr. Ken Tilson and—"

"Wait a minute," Bitsy interrupting. "Isn't he that cute guy in your French class, Nicole?"

Nicole nodded briskly.

"But he's in a wheelchair! How can he play tennis?"

"He can do *anything*," Mollie gushed, her eyes glowing with unabashed pride. "I was watching from the bushes—I mean, from my cover—and he's really good! He was making Cindy scramble for returns like crazy!"

"Really? How does he do it?" Bitsy asked, perplexed. "I mean, it's not like he can run all over the court."

"He didn't move much at all," Mollie countered. "Ken made Cindy do all the running. He made the ball go all over the place on her side."

"He must have really been something when he played," Nicole murmured.

"What do you mean?" Bitsy asked.

"Before his accident," Mollie explained. "He was a really hot tennis player. Magazines wrote him up and everything."

"Gee, that's too bad," Bitsy muttered, shaking

her head. "It must kill him, not to be able to play anymore."

"Hey, Mol. I almost forgot," Nicole interrupted. She dug into her purse and pulled out a long manila envelope. "I got this in the mail today. You just might be interested."

Nicole passed the bulky package over to her sister. Mollie quickly ripped it open and fanned the contents on the table.

"What is this?" Mollie asked. Then her eyes lit up and she read out loud in a triumphant voice, "The National Foundation of Wheelchair Tennis!"

"There was a segment about them on a news show weeks ago. I saw it while I was cooking dinner, and they listed an address to write for more information—so I did."

"They have tournaments and everything." Mollie squealed delightedly, poring over each brochure. "Look at this! There's going to be one in Santa Barbara a few weeks from now."

"Oh, I didn't see that," Nicole said, examining the schedule.

"I can't wait to tell him," Mollie exclaimed. "Ken will be thrilled."

"Just a minute, Mollie," Nicole said. "Don't you think you're being a little hasty?"

"What do you mean?"

"Well, doesn't it seem odd to you that Ken hasn't heard about this Wheelchair Tennis group already? I wouldn't do anything foolish if I were you."

"You just want to be the first to tell him yourself," Mollie said accusingly.

"Well, I was the one who found out about it," Nicole replied. "It seems only fair."

"No way!" Mollie protested. "You only became aware of this whole issue because I raised your consciousness, with all my organizing and stuff."

"You've been reading too many pamphlets," Nicole said with a sniff. "You're starting to sound like one."

"Well, it's true," Mollie complained. "I don't see why you should get the credit when I've done all the work."

"I think this is all *very* interesting," Bitsy interrupted smugly. "What a sight. Mollie and Nicole fighting over the same boy."

"We are not!" they both said indignantly.

Bitsy was grinning at them like the cat who ate the canary. Nicole opened her mouth to explain, then thought better of it. With a sly smile she daintily picked up her croissant and divided it in half.

"Want half, Mol?" she asked, holding out a piece to her sister.

"Thank you, Nicole," Mollie answered primly. They both took a bite and slowly turned to face Bitsy. Then, without another word, they chewed in silence.

Chapter 11

The moment Mollie entered Miss Shepherd's classroom on Monday, she knew something was up.

"The principal would like to see you in his office as soon as possible," her teacher instructed.

"Me?" Mollie squeaked. "What for?"

The rest of the students in her homeroom were staring at her, and all of a sudden she felt a little ill.

"Uh-oh, you're going to get it," Mark Sherman hissed from behind her.

Her friend, Linda, sitting across the aisle, mouthed the question, "What did you do now, Mol?"

Mollie shrugged helplessly and whispered, "I don't know."

"I suggest you take your books with you," Miss Shepherd added. "In case you're not back before the end of the period."

Oh, no! Mollie thought. Even Miss Shepherd thinks it's something bad.

She slowly gathered up her books, then looped her purse over her shoulder and walked stiffly to the front of the class. As she went down the aisle, kids on either side whispered, "Good luck!"

Miss Shepherd handed her a hall pass and patted Mollie on the shoulder. Mollie knew that this, too, was a bad omen. At the doorway, she smiled feebly back at her friend Linda and trudged into the empty corridor.

Her footsteps echoed in the endless hallway as she took the long walk to the principal's office.

"What did I do wrong?" she mumbled out loud, shaking her head. Suddenly, she screeched to a halt and gasped, then covered her mouth with her hand and fell back against a bank of lockers, remembering her crime.

Last winter, on February fourth, she had secretly skipped the final classes of the day. Mollie had known it was wrong, but she had had to buy her Dad a birthday present.

She started walking again, but this time a little slower and a lot more stiffly as her future passed before her eyes. As usual, she took it to the extreme, envisioning herself expelled from school. Mollie's eyes started to tear up as she imagined having to face her family after they received a call from the principal.

The office door loomed before her. She gulped and timidly pushed it open.

"Mollie Lewis?"

A lady in wire-rimmed glasses was speaking to her. She was seated at the reception desk, shuffling some papers.

"Yes, ma'am?" Mollie could hardly talk. Her lower lip was starting to quiver and she squinched her face up tight, trying not to cry.

"I'll tell the principal you're here." The woman pushed the intercom button, announced Mollie's name, and said, "Go right in."

Mollie turned to face the principal's office and was certain she heard drums, beating out a rhythm for the condemned approaching the gallows. Then she realized it was only her heart.

She stepped gingerly into the room and stood by the door, clutching her books to her chest.

Mr. Marshall was talking on the phone and gestured for her to take a seat. Mollie perched on the edge of the wooden chair in front of his desk, resigned to her fate.

When he hung up the phone she couldn't contain herself any longer. "I'm sorry, Mr. Marshall," she burst out, "for whatever I did, and I promise it won't ever happen again."

He stared at her for a moment in amazement. Then a slow smile crossed his face. "Don't you know why you're here?" he asked.

Mollie was confused and could only mutter, "No, but I can guess."

"Well," Mr. Marshall said, folding his hands on the desk in front of him and leaning forward, "it's about your letter to the school board."

"Oh." Mollie moved to the edge of her seat.

"Yes," he continued, "they were quite impressed. In fact, I understand you have been circulating a petition as well."

Mollie nodded.

"Well, I talked to Mr. Cunningham on the board this morning. He thinks it would be a good idea if you brought the petition to the next meeting on Thursday and presented it in person."

"What?" Mollie shrieked, jumping up. "They want me to what?"

Mr. Marshall laughed and said, "They would like you to speak about the difficulties disabled people face in our community." He lowered his voice confidentially. "You know, of course, that according to state law, all public buildings, including the community pool, are supposed to be accessible to every citizen. The board was shocked to discover that some are not."

"It is shocking, isn't it?" Mollie commented, her old confidence reasserting itself.

"Well," he asked, raising one eyebrow, "what do you say?"

"Gosh," she stammered, "I guess I have to say yes." Then the enormousness of the situation hit Mollie and she began to babble excitedly. "Boy, wait till my sisters hear about this! They won't believe it! They're usually the ones in the spotlight."

Mr. Marshall smiled at her enthusiasm. "Well, Mollie, you should be very proud of yourself. Your energy and dedication on this project have been quite impressive."

"Thank you, sir." Mollie smiled graciously.

Then she suddenly giggled and moved closer to the principal's desk. "You know what? I thought you had called me in here because I skipped some classes last winter—"

Her hand flew to her mouth as she realized she'd accidentally confessed right to the principal. "I mean, it was for a good reason," she added hurriedly.

Mr. Marshall tried to look stern, but his eyes were twinkling as he said, "Well, just make sure it doesn't happen again."

"Oh, no sir. It won't." Mollie quickly turned towards the door. It was time to get out of there before she revealed any more incriminating secrets.

But before she left, she turned back and asked, "Oh, one more thing. Can my family and friends come to the meeting?"

"Of course they can," Mr. Marshall said. "In fact, I would encourage you to bring all of your supporters with you."

With shoulders back and chin held high, a more confident and self-assured Mollie marched back to class. Having received the principal's blessing, she immediately began to draw up a mental list of whom to invite.

She'd have to work fast. With the French party on Wednesday and her certain triumph at the meeting on Thursday, she had a lot of phone calls to make.

That night, Nicole sat on her bed and carefully reviewed her checklist for the party. All week long she and Ken had rummaged around Santa Barbara, collecting props for the salon decor. Nicole felt confident that they were ready.

A loud squeal of delight from Mollie's room shook the rafters. Nicole heard footsteps climbing the stairs, and then her father called out, "Mollie, please! I know you're excited, but that time you broke the sound barrier."

"Sorry, Dad," Mollie yelled from her room. "I'll keep it down."

The quiet lasted for a few minutes. Then another shriek rocked the house. In spite of all the noise, Nicole couldn't keep from smiling. Ever since dinner, Mollie had been monopolizing the phone, dialing her friends and bellowing the big news about the school board.

Nicole's thoughts were interrupting by a rapping on her door.

"Who is it?" Nicole called, carefully replacing the cap on her pen.

"It's me." Cindy stuck her head around the door and crossed her eyes. "Ol' Grumpy."

Nicole laughed, pleased to see her sister coming out of her funk. When Cindy began to joke about things, Nicole knew everything would be okay.

"I wanted to apologize for being such a jerk lately," Cindy began, hovering uncertainly by the door.

"Come in and sit down," Nicole invited, motioning with her hand.

Cindy smiled sheepishly and sat down on the bed. "I guess I've been having a crisis."

"Is it over?"

Cindy squinted one eye shut and thought about it for a moment. "Not yet. But maybe I can handle it better. It's just that Liz Wright has got me tied up in knots."

"I wish I could help," Nicole offered sincerely. "Is there anything I can do?"

Cindy shook her head. "Naw, this is something I've got to work out for myself."

Another loud squawk erupted from Mollie's room, and they both jumped, then burst out laughing. Cindy leaned forward and said, "Actually there is one thing you could do."

"What's that?"

"Next time you want to know where I am, or what I'm up to—just ask me, okay? Don't put Mollie the Super Sleuth on my tail."

"Sorry," Nicole said, covering her eyes with embarrassment. "That got a little out of hand. I asked her to see what you were doing and make sure you were okay, and the next thing I know, she's in complete disguise, making a fool of herself all over town."

"That's Mollie for you." Cindy stated matter-of-factly. "She always does everything two hundred percent. Like this petition. Whoever would have thought she'd be talking to the school board?"

"Isn't it great? I'm so proud of her," Nicole said. "I just wish I could help her out with last-minute signature gathering. But I'm up to my ears with this French project."

"She doesn't seem to need our help," Cindy said. "Hardly seems like the same Mollie anymore. Maybe she's finally growing up."

Another loud shriek, stratospherically pitched, erupted from Mollie's room, and Nicole said, "Care to bet on that?"

"What's going *on* in there?" Cindy asked. "I can't take it anymore. Let's go see."

Nicole nodded, and the two of them tiptoed down the hall to Mollie's room. The door was ajar, and they could see her lying face down on the bed, with her legs kicked up behind her and her head hanging over the side. Her address book was spread out on the floor in front of her, surrounded by empty soda cans. A plate of cookies was balanced precariously beside her on the bedspread.

"She looks like she's in seventh heaven," Nicole whispered. Cindy nodded and they both turned an attentive ear to Mollie's conversation.

"Isn't it exciting, Keith?" Mollie giggled into the phone. "I mean, I was totally floored!" She twisted the cord around her finger. "Well, it is important, and because of that, I'm asking all the kids at Vista High to show up and show their support."

A male voice sounded tinnily from the receiver, and Mollie squealed. 'Oh, Keith, that's fabulous! It's this Thursday, the day after the big French party."

"What?" Nicole jerked her head up with a start, nearly hitting Cindy on the chin.

"Oh, haven't you heard?" Mollie burbled on. "Well, it's my sister Nicole's project for French class. Everyone thinks it's a great idea."

"Everyone?" Nicole repeated, getting a sinking feeling in her stomach.

"Now, don't worry," Cindy whispered soothingly, pulling Nicole away from the door. "She's too caught up in her own plans. Your party will go just the way you wanted."

Nicole listened again and breathed a sigh of relief as she overheard Mollie say, "Well, I think they are totally wrong for each other. Besides, Jason is after Claudia. Everybody knows that."

This time Cindy whispered, "Jason? Claudia? Who are they?" She knelt down to hear better, but Nicole grabbed her and pulled her away toward the staircase.

"How about some popcorn and hot chocolate?" she suggested. "Let's leave Mollie to her victory celebration."

"Aw, Nicole!" Cindy protested. "It was just getting good."

"We agreed," Nicole chastised. "No more spying."

"You are so strict," Cindy kidded, punching her sister lightly on the shoulder.

Nicole laughed, then covered her mouth with her hand. *"Mon Dieu!* I almost forgot! Cindy, would you start the popcorn? I just remembered some more things I have to add to my list for the party."

"Sure," Cindy called, leaping down the stairs.

Curiously hushed tones coming from Mollie's room made Nicole prick up her ears.

"Hi, you don't know me," Mollie whispered. "But I'm Cindy Lewis's sister."

Nicole hesitated, fighting the urge to eavesdrop.

It's none of my business, she thought, and stepped briskly down the hall to her room.

Chapter 12

On the evening of the party, the front doorbell rang just as Nicole was putting the last touches on her costume.

"I'll get it," she sang out merrily, and floated down the stairs in her shimmering white tutu. The skirt and petticoat came to just below her knees and rustled coolly as she walked. She had sewn multicolored ribbons onto the pink ballet slippers on her feet and laced them around her calves.

Nicole had chosen to host the party as a ballet dancer from a painting by Degas. With her hair tied into a tight bun on the top of her head and a black satin ribbon around her neck, she looked as though she could've stepped right off the painter's canvas.

At the foot of the stairs her nerves got the better of her confidence and she surveyed the living room with a critical eye.

Everything seemed to be in order. The windows were hung with heavy red velvet drapes, on loan from the Vista High theater department. The little round café tables her mother had borrowed from Le Bistro were laden with delectable hors d'oeuvres.

Satisfied that all was it should be, Nicole took a deep breath and opened the door, only to be greeted with a huge bouquet of wildflowers.

"Bon soir, mademoiselle!" a voice crooned from behind the bouquet. "These are for you. *Des belles fleurs* for a lovely flower."

Nicole graciously accepted the bouquet and then laughed with delight when she saw Ken's disguise.

"Toulouse-Lautrec," Nicole burst out. "Oh, Ken, you look absolutely perfect."

He was wearing a black satin cape with a theatrical purple lining. A dashing velvet cravat was wrapped around the old-fashioned wing collar of his white shirt, which disappeared into a hounds-tooth-check vest. A derby sat on his head at a rakish tilt and a pair of pince-nez teetered on the bridge of his nose.

As she inhaled the lovely scent of the bouquet, Ken swung his wheelchair toward the doorjamb and said, "May I come in?"

"Oh! Of course," Nicole answered, throwing the

door wide open. *"Entrez, s'il vous plaît."* Ken maneuvered the chair over the bump and rolled easily into the living room.

"One thing about your house, Nicole"—he grinned—"nice level entryway. I just hate split-level houses."

"Oh, Ken," Nicole whispered, nervously gripping his hand, "I'm so nervous."

Ken pressed her palm reassuringly. "Relax, Nicole. Everything looks—*comment on dit?* How you say? *Magnifique!*"

"Well, I've checked and double-checked everything, including the guest list, which, I'm embarrassed to say, has grown to twenty people."

"That's not too bad," Ken assured her. "I'm sure Madame Preston won't mind a few extra people. Should liven up our salon a bit."

Nicole bit her lip anxiously. "I just wish my sisters had consulted me first before they handed out the invitations."

"Where are they, anyway?" Ken asked, pushing open the kitchen door and peering inside. "Aren't they supposed to act as our official greeters?"

"They're upstairs in Mom's room. She's helping them with their costumes. Grant and Duffy are around here, too, somewhere."

Just then Duffy appeared at the top of the stairs, whistling the French national anthem, the "Marseillaise." He was wearing a gray painter's smock, with a floppy green beret on his head. He had drawn on a beard with a red lip liner, and his left ear was covered with a bizarre bandage of gauze and surgical tape.

At the same moment Grant threw open the kitchen door and stepped to the foot of the stairs.

"Ta-da!" he crowed, opening his arms to accept their applause.

Then he saw Duffy. Their costumes were almost identical, down to the beret and the bandaged left ear. They stared at each other, aghast, and bellowed, "Vince!"

Duffy came down the steps, shaking his head. "And I thought I was being so original. . . ."

"Me, too," Grant echoed, grinning at Nicole and Ken. "Maybe I should have come as Paul Goggin."

"Who?" Nicole asked, unfamiliar with the name. Her mind was still reeling with the horrible specter of multiple Vincent Van Goghs.

"You know, Van Gogh's buddy," Grant continued. "The guy that went off to Tahiti and never came back."

Ken and Nicole burst our laughing at the same time. "You mean, Paul Gauguin," Ken explained. "It's pronounced 'Go-*ganh*.' "

"*Bonsoir,* everybody!" Mollie trilled from the top of the stairs, interrupting their impromptu lesson. She spun in a little circle to show off her costume. Pink and white roses were pinned to the bodice of her long blue dress and echoed the brightly colored splash of a hat on her head.

"Who are you?" Nicole asked.

Mollie gave her a smugly superior look. "The

flower seller in Renoir's *On the Terrace*" she pronounced. "Don't you ever look at your Impressionist calendar? I'm the month of April."

Mollie was so busy showing off that she hadn't noticed Duffy standing nearby. When she did she gasped in horror. "Duffy, what did you do to your ear?"

"Nozing," he said in a terrible French accent. "Zis eez pahrt of mon cos-*toom*!" Then, in his normal voice, he explained. "After Vince had a fight with his friend, Gauguin," he said, "he sliced off his ear and mailed it to his girlfriend."

"Oh, gross!" Mollie shrieked, wrinkling her nose. "If anyone ever did that to me, I'd *never* speak to him again."

"She didn't," Ken cracked.

"Battle stations, everybody," Cindy shouted, bursting out of her room. "Four cars just pulled into our driveway."

She skipped down the stairs, still fastening a big bow at the neck of her painter's smock, and charged past Ken and Nicole into the kitchen. She was wearing a long gray beard made out of construction paper and string.

"Who's she supposed to be?" Mollie asked.

"Renoir, of course" came the reply from the kitchen.

Niçole fluttered over to the stereo and slipped a cassette into the tape machine. As delicate strains of music by Claude Debussy filled the air, Duffy and Grant took their positions by the door. Ken wheeled over to an easel they had placed in the corner of the living room. As soon as everyone was in position, Nicole sang out, "Let's begin!"

The front doorbell rang, and Duffy threw open the door with a flourish. "*Bonsoir* and—*what?*"

There, standing on the steps, was a tall guy in a gorilla mask and short guy grinning from behind Groucho Marx glasses-nose-and-mustache.

"Hey! It's my man!" the gorilla cried out, then yelled over his shoulder. "It's Duffy. We've come to the right place."

The short guy explained, "Mollie Lewis said there was going to be a big costume party here. Hey, look at all that food!"

Before Duffy could respond, the two guys headed straight for the hors d'oeuvres. Nicole and Ken watched open-mouthed as five more uninvited guests in masks and strange costumes sailed through the door.

Within the next hour their intimate "Paris salon" was packed with a noisy crowd of chattering kids, most of whom had never heard of the Impressionists. They stood around talking in phony French and raving about what a great party it was.

At first Nicole tried to make the best of it. But the sight of an appalled Madame Preston, staring at the chaos around her, convinced Nicole that the event was a disaster.

Biting back her tears, Nicole rushed up the

stairs to her room and threw herself in a hopeless clump onto her bed.

Meanwhile Cindy was frantically ransacking the kitchen, trying to find something to put out on the tables to eat. The hors d'oeuvres had disappeared in the first hour, and the cheese and crackers were almost gone. She held a half-empty jar of sweet pickles in front of her face and toyed with the idea of putting them in a bowl.

"Bleagh! I hate pickles." She grimaced, setting them back on the shelf. Then she spied an almost full carton of sour cream.

"A dip! That's the ticket!" In a flash she had an armful of herbs and spices spread out on the kitchen counter, ready to be whipped into a snappy concoction. But then her inspiration failed her.

"Where's Nicole?" she grumbled. "She'd know how to make something good out of this. It's her party, anyway. Why am *I* doing this?"

"Uh—Cindy?"

At the sound of her name, Cindy whirled around and found herself staring straight into the eye of her rival, Liz Wright.

"I—I wanted to thank you for inviting me to the party," the girl began hesitantly. "I'm having a great time!"

Cindy's jaw fell open and she just stood there, thunderstruck. Liz Wright was the last person on earth she'd invite to a party. What was she talking about?

"This is the first time I've had a chance to really meet anybody here in Santa Barbara," Liz said with a shy smile. "I really appreciate the gesture."

Cindy finally found her voice. "Sure. Anytime."

After an awkward silence, Liz started to leave the room. Then she turned and said, "Oh, about the coaching sessions. I'd be happy to help you, anytime."

Cindy felt like she'd been slapped in the face. "What are you talking about?" she asked, her voice tight in her throat.

Liz's smile faded. "When Mollie called with your invitation, she said that you wanted me to help you with your stroke."

At the mention of Mollie's name, a bell went off in Cindy's brain. Of course. Who else would do such a dumb thing? Her mind was almost numb with shock.

"That's right, isn't it?"

The sound of Liz's voice jolted Cindy back to the present. Liz was staring at her, an uncertain, almost hurt look in her eyes. In a flash Cindy realized that Liz had been sincere. She was also a guest in the Lewis home and deserved to be treated politely. Which was not, however, how Cindy intended to treat Mollie once she got a hold of her.

"Oh, sure," Cindy said, plastering on what she hoped was a pleasant smile. "How thoughtful of Mollie to call you." She took a deep breath. "Where is my sister, anyway?" she asked sweetly, her face a careful mask of politeness. "Have you seen her?"

After Liz shook her head, Cindy managed to excuse herself and get out of the kitchen before her face revealed what she was really thinking.

"Hey, where's the dip?" Duffy asked, coming up beside her, a potato chip in his hand.

"Where's Mollie?" Cindy demanded, ignoring him. "I have to—" Cindy stopped in mid-sentence when she spotted Mollie out on the patio, surrounded by her costumed friends.

"Never mind," Cindy muttered grimly, her eyes locked on her sister. "I've found her."

"Nicole?" a voice called from outside the bedroom door. "It's me, Bitsy. Can I come in?"

Nicole raised her head off the damp pillow and murmured weakly, *"Oui. Entrez."*

Bitsy was the only friend outside of French class that Nicole had invited. At least she had taken their project seriously. She had come dressed as the painter Mary Cassatt.

"Everyone's asking about you!" Bitsy whispered, sitting down next to her friend on the bed. "What are you doing up here?"

"Hiding," Nicole moaned, rolling over onto her back. The lace net from her tutu spread out around her body like a paper fan.

"Why? The party is a huge success. Everyone's having a great time."

"Bitsy, this isn't a party! It's a project for class.

We were trying to recreate a Paris salon of the 1880s. Everyone was to dress as an artist or figure from that time. And everyone was supposed to speak French."

"Well, a lot of people are trying their darnedest," Bitsy said with a giggle. "I think 'Frere Jacques' has been sung at least ten times."

"That's what I mean," Nicole wailed. "It's just a big free-for-all down there. And hardly anyone is in costume.

"Now, that's not true," Bitsy broke in. "Granted some people didn't arrive in costume, but now they're all wearing something."

"What do you mean?"

"I saw Mollie handing out ski caps and tams to the newcomers. They tried to make them look like berets."

"You're kidding!" Nicole gasped in horror.

"No, I'm not, and I think everyone is wearing a mustache," Bitsy said. "That girl, Heather—you know, she's in all the plays at Vista—she appointed herself makeup artist and she's drawing them on anyone who will sit still."

"Oh, it's worse than I thought." Nicole clutched her stomach and groaned. "I bet Madame Preston is long gone."

"No, she's still here. I saw her talking to the water-polo team by the fireplace."

Nicole's eyes started to fill with tears. "We worked so hard on this. Researching the Impressionists, and the Neo-, and Post-Impressionists.

Ken and I were even going to give a little lecture about it, all in French."

"Well, Ken's been giving his and it's really funny, especially when Duffy tries to translate. They've kept everyone in stitches."

"He must think I'm just awful for deserting him," Nicole said, wiping her eyes with a tissue.

"I don't think he's noticed. He's been too busy giving his speech and painting portraits."

"I didn't know Ken could paint," Nicole said sitting up.

"He can't," Bitsy said. "But it's the thought that counts."

Nicole tried to join in the laughter, but the sound died in her throat as she thought once more about "what might have been."

"Oooh." Nicole pummeled the bed with her fist. "I could just strangle Mollie! She has totally ruined our project."

"Well, if you're really upset, you should do something about it," Bitsy observed reasonably.

"Like what?" Nicole asked.

"Like, tell people to leave."

Nicole covered her head with the pillow. "I couldn't. I'd be too embarrassed."

Bitsy picked up the edge of the pillow and ordered, "Then make Mollie do it."

Nicole jerked her head out and looked directly at her friend. "I should!" she declared. "After all, I'm the one who's going to get a big, fat *F* on this, not her." Her feeling of total defeat was transforming into righteous indignation. "It'd serve her right, having to embarrass herself in front of everybody."

"That's the spirit!" Bitsy clapped her hands with glee. "For a minute there, I thought you'd turned into Camille."

Nicole hopped off the bed and checked herself in the mirror on the back of the door. After wiping away the smudged mascara and dabbing a little powder under her eyes, she felt ready for battle.

A determined Nicole flung open her door and marched down the stairs, with Bitsy close on her heels.

She knew exactly what to do. First she would find Ken and apologize for her desertion. And then she would lower the boom on Mollie the Meddler.

Chapter 13

"*Attention, everybody!*" Mollie called to the crowd that had gathered on the back patio. "*Ah—tenh-cion!*" she cried again, giving the word a French pronunciation. Her cheeks were flushed with excitement. For some reason Nicole and Cindy had vanished, so she was beginning to feel that this was her party—hers and Ken's.

"*Bonjour,* everybody!" Mollie began, waving her hand merrily. The group echoed, "*Bonjour!*" right back at her, and a couple of the guys struck up an impromptu chorus of "*Alouette.*" Duffy and Grant managed to get them to quiet down, and finally the group turned toward Mollie expectantly. She hopped up on a cane-backed chair and anxiously scanned the crowd. There was still no sign of Cindy and Nicole.

"I have a big announcement to make," she explained, "but I want my sisters, and Ken, to hear it. Has anybody seen them?"

A loud buzzing went around the group until finally a voice near the sliding glass doors called out, "Here they are!"

Off to her right, Mollie could see Ken wheel his chair through the kitchen door and stop near the rosebushes. The patio lights created a glare on the sliding glass doors, but Mollie was just able to make out her sisters.

"First of all, I'd like to say welcome from the entire Lewis family. I know my sisters want to add their—" She turned to look at Nicole and Cindy and immediately her huge grin turned into a look of shock.

Mollie gasped. For some reason, her sisters didn't seem too happy. In fact, they looked downright mad. Cindy was heading right for her with her arms crossed and her jaw clenched. Right behind her came Nicole, and she wasn't smiling, either. The crowd seemed to part before them, creating a path that led directly to Mollie.

What could be wrong with them? Mollie wondered. This party's going so well. What could they possibly have to be so mad about? Then it occurred to her. Her sisters must be jealous that she was the star of the show for once. Well, she wasn't about to give ground now. The diminutive blonde drew herself up to her full height and addressed the crowd.

"I'd like to thank each and every one of you for signing my petition and for your support on this drive," Mollie called out. "We've gotten nearly six hundred signatures, and I know that will make a big impression on the school board when I give it to them tomorrow night!"

The group surged closer to Mollie, clapping and whistling their approval.

She was elated by their response. A jolt of energy shot up her spine as she realized she felt just like Norma Rae, rallying the workers to her cause.

"That brings me to my big announcement," she continued, when the applause had settled down. "It's about our friend Ken Tilson." She gestured grandly toward Ken, who looked surprised but waved genially as everybody looked his way. "Some of you may not know this, but before his accident, Ken was a great tennis player." An impressed murmur rippled through the audience. "And I'm sure he still is. Just because you're in a wheelchair doesn't mean you're not an athlete anymore. And to prove it, Ken will be representing Vista High in the men's singles of the National Foundation of Wheelchair Tennis Tournament, which takes place here in Santa Barbara two weeks from today!"

This time the roar was deafening. As Mollie led the cheering, well-wishers swarmed around Ken, clapping him on the back and shaking his hand.

Mollie looked over at him proudly to catch his reaction.

Ken was sitting absolutely stock-still. The smile had completely faded from his face and he stared in disbelief at Mollie. His jaw was taut with fury, and she thought the anger in his eyes would burn a hole through her.

An awkward silence settled upon the crowd as they waited for the next announcement. Mollie was too stunned to go on. Her confidence was completely shattered, and her confusion was obvious.

Quickly Nicole sprang into action. She tugged Mollie by the sleeve and whispered, "Get down this instant! I'll handle this."

Mollie started to protest, but Nicole abruptly yanked her off the chair, whispering, "I think you've done enough damage, Mollie." Then she climbed up and onto the chair and raised her arms to get everyone's attention.

"*Mesdames et messieurs!* There are fresh croissants and pastries in the dining room, courtesy of my mother's catering business, Movable Feast."

Nicole directed them all back inside the house as she called out, "*Bon appétit!*"

Within moments the patio was deserted. It was with a sinking dread that Mollie realized that she was alone with her sisters and Ken.

"How could you?" Nicole was the first to ask the question that was on everyone's lips. "What was going on in your mind? What could possibly have convinced you that what you were doing was right?"

"What do you mean?" Mollie asked timidly. She was pretty confused as to what they were all so upset about. Her response sent Cindy and Nicole both off at once.

"You ... you ..." Nicole stammered in her anger. "You just take things into your own hands!"

"You make decisions for other people without even asking them!" Cindy fumed.

"How could you invite all those other people to this party," Nicole continued, "when you *knew* this was my project for school? I mean the *whole* water-polo team?"

"I didn't actually invite them," Mollie corrected feebly. "I just happened to mention your party when I was calling everyone with my good news. Then the word just kind of spread, I guess."

"How could you have told Liz that I invited her?" Cindy demanded. "Of all the people—"

"This whole party has been nothing but a complete and total disaster," Nicole said, cutting her off.

"That's not true, Nicole," Cindy objected. "I mean it's not what you planned, but I'd say it's a big success."

"Thanks, Cin," Mollie peeped, grateful for Cindy's defense.

"No thanks to you," Cindy barked at her, her glare leaving no doubt that Mollie was still in the doghouse.

"Well, whatever you call it," Nicole raised her voice, "it means a failing grade or a completely new project."

"Who ever gave you the right to invite Liz, anyway?" Cindy said, resuming her attack on Mollie. "And then, adding insult to injury, you told her I wanted lessons from her. I don't believe you!"

"All of this work for nothing," Nicole moaned. Both girls circled Mollie shaking their heads in frustration.

Suddenly all three of them realized that throughout their squabbling, Ken hadn't uttered a word. He sat in his chair, not looking at them, his eyes fixed on the ground.

"Ken," Mollie asked in a shaky voice, "aren't you going to yell at me, too?"

He looked up at her and shook his head. "No. I don't think yelling would do any good."

"You aren't mad at me, then?"

"I'm beyond mad," Ken said, his voice under control. "I'm in shock." He took off his derby and beard and lowered them to his lap, then stared down at his hands. After a moment he took a deep breath and said, "You see, Mollie, I didn't really mind when you, uh, adopted me as your personal cause. Because I liked you and your family, and I thought, well, what harm could it do?" He cleared his throat. "But I never expected it to go this far. Most people who start off with good intentions rarely follow them through to the end." He smiled at her ruefully. "You surprised me. But even so, this petition, the speech to the school board, it can only help disabled people as a whole. So I didn't mind."

All three girls held their breath, waiting for his next sentence.

"But today you crossed the line," he went on. "You interfered with my personal life. And you had no business doing that."

"Ken, that's not what I meant to do," Mollie responded earnestly. "I thought you would love to play tennis again."

"I'll decide if and when I play tennis." His voice was tight.

"And when will that be?" Cindy asked boldly.

Ken shot her a surprised look and answered, "When I feel I'm ready."

"You're ready now," Cindy blurted out. There was no mistaking the challenge in her voice, and Ken stiffened visibly.

She said quickly, "Look, I know Mollie had no right entering you in the competition without your permission. But I think you should do it."

"Who asked you?" Ken snapped.

"I'm just giving my opinion," Cindy replied. "Because I know you could compete."

"Yeah," Nicole chimed in. "Cindy told us what a mean backhand you have."

"And when I saw you play, I thought you looked great," Mollie added.

"What is this, a conspiracy?" Ken exploded. "Stop trying to run my life, all three of you!"

There was a shocked silence. His words stung Nicole and Mollie, but Cindy was not about to be dismayed.

"What are you afraid of?" she demanded. "Not winning? Being made a fool of? That maybe you aren't the best anymore?"

Ken jerked up his head to reply but Cindy cut him off. "You'll never know until you try. Until you give it your best shot. You're standing in your own way, your only enemy is yourself."

Her words sounded strangely familiar, and with a start she remembered where she'd heard them before. Ken had tried to tell her exactly the same thing about her swimming.

The air seemed electrified with tension. Ken clutched the rims of his wheels until his knuckles turned white. Finally he spoke.

"My life was just going fine until I met the three of you. I got along without you in the past," he said hoarsely, "and I'll do just fine without you in the future."

He spun his chair around to the side exit of the patio, stopping to throw open the little gate. Then he turned and looked at Nicole.

"Please express my regrets to Madame Preston," he said stiffly, "and the rest of our class."

Without waiting for a response, Ken wheeled around the side of the house and disappeared into the darkness.

The three girls stood side by side, stunned into silence. All the color had drained from Mollie's face. Nicole suddenly felt dizzy and had to put her hand on the back of the chair for support.

Cindy stared intently in the direction Ken had gone. She muttered something under her breath.

"What did you say?" Nicole asked.

Cindy glanced over and said gruffly, "I said he could win."

"Look, Cindy, it's time to drop it," Nicole said firmly. "I think we've interfered enough in Ken's life."

"Yeah," Mollie said softly. "Poor Ken."

Cindy and Nicole were suddenly reminded of all Mollie's crimes, and they both turned on her at once.

"Listen, shrimp," Cindy began. "We're not through with you yet. Tomorrow night, when you go to that board meeting, you're on your own."

"Oh, no, my speech!" Mollie gasped. "Ken was supposed to go over it with me."

"Well, I think you can safely assume that won't be happening," Nicole said. "In fact, I would be very surprised if Ken Tilson ever spoke to any one of us again."

At that moment the partygoers inside struck up another rousing chorus of "Alouette." The cheerful singing seemed out of place now.

"I've got to go back inside," Nicole said quietly.

"I'm still the hostess. I have to see this through to the end."

With just the hint of tears in her eyes, she turned away from her sisters and entered the house.

Chapter 14

"Will somebody help me, please!"

Mollie stood at the top of the stairs and shouted down to the living room. The Lewis house was in an uproar. It was a quarter to seven on Thursday evening. The school board meeting, the most important event of Mollie's life, would begin in just forty-five minutes, and she was absolutely paralyzed with fear. She stood in her slip, wearing one shoe and holding three different dresses.

"Mollie, get dressed," her father shouted up at her from the foot of the stairs.

"But, Daddy, I don't have anything to wear," she wailed.

"Mollie, if you don't get dressed in the next five minutes, I'm taking you there in your underwear," he replied.

One thing Mr. Lewis insisted on was punctuality.

"Now, Richard," Mrs. Lewis chastened, coming into the hall, "you're only making Mollie more nervous by rushing her. I'm sure she'll be ready on time."

"I guess I'm a little jumpy myself," he said, rubbing his hand over his bald spot. "But where *is* everybody, anyway? Where's Nicole? And Cindy? Why aren't they home yet?"

"Now, calm down, dear," Mrs. Lewis said soothingly, guiding Mr. Lewis into the living room. At the foot of the stairs, she called, "Mollie, I'll be right up."

Her last word was drowned out by the bang of Mollie's door as she slammed it shut. She slumped miserably on the edge of her bed. How was she ever going to survive the night?

The past twenty-four hours had been complete agony, with everyone shunning her. Last night she'd gone straight to her room and cried herself to sleep. Her sisters completely ignored her at breakfast, and then when neither of them came home for dinner she knew she was on her own.

She choked back a sob and thought of Ken. That hurt look in his eyes had haunted her all night. She was sure he'd never forgive her. Everything seemed so hopeless. It didn't even seem worth it to be giving her speech anymore. Just when Mollie was about to burst into tears, the door swung open and Mollie turned, preparing to sob on her mother's shoulder. Instead she saw her sister silhouetted in the doorway.

"Nicole?" she whispered. "I thought Mom—"

"She's got her hands full with Dad downstairs," Nicole said briskly, crossing to Mollie and yanking her to her feet. "Here, put this on."

Mollie, stunned with surprise, obediently held her arms above her head.

"Nicole, you don't have to help me," she mumbled. "I'd understand if you didn't."

The feel of rich silk traveling over her body brought Mollie to her senses.

"Oh, Nicole, this is your new blouse," she cried. "I can't possibly wear it."

"Yes, you can," Nicole replied. "Now put on that gray linen skirt you just bought." As soon as Mollie had pulled on her skirt, Nicole dragged her to the full-length mirror on the back of the door. "See how elegant you look?"

Mollie gasped at her reflection. The silk blouse was a lovely cornflower blue and it brought out the color of her eyes. It draped beautifully across the shoulders and narrowed at the waist. She looked mature and beautiful, and almost grown-up.

She looked over her shoulder at her sister and asked hesitantly, "Does this mean you're not mad at me?"

Nicole took a deep breath. "It means that you're my sister and I love you, and I want you to look and do your best tonight." Then she added, "Because whatever you do reflects on all of us."

Mollie's chin started to quiver and her eyes brimmed with tears.

"And no, I'm not still mad at you," Nicole said gently.

"Oh, Nicole, I'm so happy!" Mollie yelled, wrapping her arms around her sister and almost knocking her over. "I couldn't bear it if you hated me."

"But, if you *ever* pull something like that again ..."

"Never, never again. I promise."

They hugged each other tightly for a moment. Then Nicole snatched up a tissue and tried to salvage Mollie's makeup.

"Nicole, I'm so nervous." Mollie held a trembling arm out in front of her. "Look at my hand. I'll never be able to give my speech. The paper will shake too much."

"Nonsense," Nicole said, quickly brushing out Mollie's hair. "I'm sure there will be a podium for you to stand behind. They're very good for disguising shaking knees and hands."

The news about the podium made Mollie feel a little better, but not much. She took three deep breaths and tried to relax.

"Your mother and I are leaving, Mollie. Are you coming?" Mr. Lewis shouted up the stairs.

Mollie shrieked.

"Better hurry, honey," Mrs. Lewis said. "Your father is getting impatient."

"We'll be right down," Nicole promised.

As they came down the stairs, Mollie walking very slowly and gripping the handrail in her nervousness, Winston greeted them and nearly knocked them both over in his excitement. Outside, their father was already behind the steering wheel honking the horn.

"Oh, Nicole," Mollie said suddenly, clutching her sister's hand. "I wish Cindy were coming. It would make everything perfect. Besides"—she gulped nervously—"I need all the support I can get."

"She'll be there," Nicole assured her confidently.

Mrs. Lewis appeared in the front door. "If you don't get in the car right now, I'm afraid we'll never make it on time."

Nicole gathered up the petition and Mollie's speech from the table by the door, and the sisters charged for the waiting car.

"Now, the important thing," Mr. Lewis cautioned, "is to remain calm." His foot hit the accelerator and the car screeched off down the street.

The meeting was being held in the multipurpose room of Lowell Junior High. As the car neared the school, Mollie noticed two figures standing on the sidewalk out front.

"Look, everybody!" Mollie shouted, bouncing up and down in her seat. "Cindy's here!"

"Who's that other girl with her?" Mrs. Lewis asked, flipping down the overhead mirror and checking her lipstick one last time.

"I'm not sure," Nicole said, leaning across Mollie to peer out the window. "She doesn't look familiar."

But Mollie recognized her. It was Liz Wright.

Now she didn't know what to do. Butterflies started flying around in her stomach. They wouldn't both yell at her, would they?

"Everybody jump out here," Mr. Lewis ordered, "and meet me at the front door."

They got out of the car and joined Cindy and her companion on the sidewalk.

"Cindy, we were worried about you," Laura Lewis admonished her daughter gently, giving her a quick hug.

"Sorry, Mom, I know I should've called. I had a private coaching session today after practice." Cindy gestured to the girl standing a few feet behind her, clad in jeans and a warm-up jacket. "With Liz."

"Oh, you're the swimmer I've heard so much about," Mrs. Lewis said, shaking her hand.

"Lizzie's a *great* swimmer," Cindy corrected. "Her father is a coach. She's been in training since she was seven."

"Yeah," Liz joked. "Dad threw all of us in the pool when we were little and hasn't let us out since. I don't think he'll be happy until we grow gills."

"I thought you already had them," Cindy kidded.

"Not yet," Liz shot back. "but I wouldn't be surprised if you did." Then she turned to Mrs. Lewis. "You should be really proud of your daughter, Mrs. Lewis. She's a natural."

"Hello, Liz," Nicole said, offering her hand. "I'm Nicole. Cindy's older sister."

"I know," Liz grinned. "I was at your French party yesterday. Mollie invited me."

"Oh, that's right." Nicole nodded. Then she raised an eyebrow toward Mollie. "She invited a lot of people. Part of her little plan to help out."

Mollie squeezed her eyes shut, waiting for the lecture she was dreading. To her surprise, Cindy came up and draped her arm around her shoulders.

"Well, in my case, shrimp, it worked out!"

"Huh?" Mollie opened her eyes wide and stared at her sister.

"Liz and I made a deal," Cindy explained. "She coaches me on my swimming and I teach her to surf."

"Oh, Cindy." Mollie jumped up and down. "That's great!"

"Yeah," Cindy said. "Lucky for you. One of your bright ideas actually worked out."

"Well, to be precise," Nicole interrupted, "two of them did."

"What do you mean?" Cindy demanded.

Nicole smiled mysteriously. "Madame Preston gave our French project an *A*."

"What?" Mollie shrieked. "You didn't tell me that!"

"I didn't want you to think you could get off the hook so easily," Nicole said pointedly. Then she explained to the others. "Madame Preston said we've created more interest in French at Vista than anything she's ever tried." She giggled and added, "People were coming in and out of her office all morning, wanting to join the French club."

"Hey!" someone shouted from across the parking lot. Mr. Lewis raced across the gravel to his family, pointing frantically at his watch as he ran.

"What are you doing out here?" he gasped. "We've only got three minutes until this thing begins!"

"Oh, no!" Mollie cried. "I've got to make a speech!"

"Oh, Richard, look what you've done!" Mrs. Lewis chided as she wrapped a comforting arm around Mollie. "You've made her nervous again."

"Sorry, Mollie," Mr. Lewis apologized, patting her arm nervously. "There's nothing to worry about. You're going to do just fine."

With Mollie firmly supported between them, Mr. and Mrs. Lewis set off resolutely toward the entrance to the auditorium.

The noise in the multipurpose room was deafening. The room was used as a cafeteria during the day, and the lunch tables were stacked up against the walls. At one end was a large stage with a conference table set up for the board members. Chairs had been put out in rows, and people were clustered in groups along the aisles, chattering among themselves.

"Wow!" Cindy exclaimed. "It looks like half of Vista High is here!"

With glazed eyes Mollie glanced around the

crowded room and groaned, "Me and my big mouth."

"Ladies and gentlemen," a man announced from the microphone on the stage, "if you'll take your seats, this meeting will get under way."

The Lewises found an empty row of folding chairs near the back and settled into their places. There was great screeching of chairs and a rumble of chatter as the rest of the crowd did the same.

"All right," the man said, as soon as quiet was restored. "it looks like we're ready to begin. Glad to see such a terrific turnout. I'm Mike Cunningham, president of your school board, and this meeting is now called to order."

He quickly read off the agenda for the evening. Much to her dismay, Mollie discovered that her speech was scheduled close to the end.

As the secretary read the minutes from the previous session, Mollie was seized with a violent case of nerves. She leaned over to her mother and whispered, "I've got to get a drink of water, Mom. I'll be right back."

She lurched up from her seat and inched down the aisle past her father, who smiled and pointed at his watch.

Nicole looked up worriedly, as if to say, "Do you want me to come with you?" Mollie shook her head and tiptoed quickly into the hall.

Once outside in the empty corridor, she found the fountain and took a deep drink of water.

Every part of her body felt shaky. Her heart pounded loudly in her chest. Her mouth had completely dried up and her hands were vibrating a mile a minute, as though they didn't belong to her anymore.

Mollie leaned her head back against the tiled wall and clutched her stomach.

"I can't go through with this," she moaned.

A voice beside her calmly replied, "Of course you can."

Chapter 15

"Ken!" Mollie cried out. "You came."

"Of course I came," he replied with a smile. "I couldn't pass up the chance to see a Lewis take on the school board, could I?"

Mollie giggled with relief.

"Oh, Ken, I'm so glad you're here. I couldn't do it without—"

Mollie stopped herself, remembering how angry he'd been the day before. Then she stammered, "Well, I'm just giving a little speech. It's no big deal."

"For me it is." Ken pushed his chair closer to her and demanded, "Or have you forgotten why you're here? Why you spent all that time and energy talking to people, getting signatures, gathering support."

His forceful words startled her, and she didn't know how to respond.

Then Ken answered for her. "Because we want to attend all of Cindy's swim meets. And go into Pete's through the front door. Right?"

"Right." Mollie smiled courageously, standing up a little straighter. There was a sudden burst of applause inside the auditorium and her confidence quickly faded.

"There are so many people in there," she wailed. "Oh, Ken, I'm so nervous. I'll never make it through my speech." Her hands began to quiver again and she slumped back against the wall.

The door to the meeting room opened a crack, and Cindy whispered hoarsely into the hall. "Hey, shrimp? Are you okay? Dad's getting really nervous."

"Tell him I'll be there in time," she answered. "I'm just talking to Ken."

"Ken?" Cindy peered around the door, then stepped out into the hall and walked toward them. She stopped a little distance from Ken, a chagrined look on her face. He looked up and their eyes met.

"Hey, Cindy." He waved a hand in greeting.

"You still speaking to me?" Cindy asked, her eyes widening in surprise. "After I shot my mouth off yesterday, I was afraid you'd—"

"Hey, I thought a lot about what you said," Ken interrupted, holding up his hand. "And maybe you were right. Maybe I am my own worst enemy."

"I guess we all are." Cindy grinned. "Just look at me."

Then she whispered confidentially, "Liz and I decided to work together. And you know what? I even like her."

"Yeah?" Ken smiled up at her. "Well, I've got some news of my own." He looked over at Mollie. "I've decided to give the tournament a shot."

Mollie started to squeal with delight, but Cindy clapped a hand over her mouth and stifled it just in time. Mollie nodded her head and Cindy let go.

"That's great, Ken!" Mollie whispered.

"It is," Cindy agreed. "By the way, if you need a partner to practice with—"

"Funny you should mention it," Ken broke in. "I was just about to ask."

"Say no more," Cindy said with a laugh. "Meet me at the court on Manzanita tomorrow at four and be prepared to do battle."

"It's a deal," Ken declared as they shook on it.

"Mollie." Nicole stuck her head out into the hall. "Mollie, you're next. Come on."

When Nicole saw Ken with her sisters, her heart skipped a beat. She started to rush toward him but caught herself.

"I'm glad you came," she said formally. "I know how much Mollie appreciates your support." Then she turned to go back into the meeting.

"Wait, Nicole," Ken called after her. "I want to apologize. I said some harsh things yesterday and—"

"And we deserved them," Nicole replied.

Ken held out his hand. "Friends?"

Nicole clasped it warmly. "Friends."

All four of them froze as a voice boomed from the auditorium.

"Our next speaker will be Mollie Lewis, from Vista High."

"Oh, no. That's me," Mollie gasped."I can't do it. I don't know what ever made me think I could." She grabbed Nicole by the sleeve and desperately pleaded. "You do it for me, Nicole. I can't."

"Hold it, Mollie," Ken ordered. He turned to Cindy and Nicole and asked, "Is this the same Mollie Lewis I met by the library? Mollie the Crusader?"

Nicole and Cindy crossed their arms and stared curiously at Mollie.

"I don't know," Nicole said, shaking her head.

"It can't be," Ken scoffed.

Cindy scratched her chin and said, "You mean, the girl who brought archrivals like Cindy Lewis and Liz Wright together?"

"Who took a good idea for a French project," Nicole joined in, "and turned it into the cultural event of the year?"

"And last but not least," Ken added, raising a finger, "the girl who got an ex–tennis champ back in the game?"

"I did all that?" Mollie asked, wide-eyed.

"You sure did," Ken answered. "So what's so

hard about giving a speech in front of a few friends?"

The voice from the auditorium boomed again. "Is Mollie Lewis here?"

"Yes," Nicole shouted, throwing open the door. "She's on her way!"

"Ken!" Mollie gripped his arm tightly. "Come up there with me, please!"

He squeezed her hand and nodded. "Sure."

Nicole and Cindy swung the doors open and held them back while Ken rolled into the meeting room. Heads craned to see what the commotion was. Ken slowly wheeled his chair down the long aisle toward the stage. Mollie walked beside him, with one hand on his shoulder. She was in a bewildered daze. Nicole and Cindy followed close behind.

As Mollie passed by her parents, her mom stopped her and slipped the speech and petition under her arm. Then Mrs. Lewis kissed her daughter lightly on the cheek and gently shoved her toward the stage.

A few feet before the edge of the stage Ken stopped moving. "I don't believe it," he muttered.

"What's the matter?" Mollie whispered.

"Look," he answered, pointing at the stage.

It seemed normal enough—just a platform about three feet high hung with black drapes. There was an American flag to the left and two sets of steps on either side leading down to the floor.

"I can't get up there, Mollie," Ken said quietly. "There are no ramps."

Mollie froze with fear. She looked back up at the stage. Six important-looking people were sitting at the conference table, staring at her. She turned to Ken in anguish.

"You've got to be there!" she pleaded. "I can't do it alone!"

Ken shook his head. "You're on your own now, Mollie." He pressed her hand hard. "I'll be right here watching."

Mollie edged toward the steps, clutching her petition in her hands. She stumbled at the top and for one horrible second thought she'd lose her balance and fall. It seemed to take her hours to cover the few feet to the podium. Gratefully she grasped the sides of the lectern and took her first glance at the audience.

Everywhere Mollie looked, upturned faces gazed back at her, waiting expectantly to hear what she had come to say. Mollie lowered the microphone to her own petite height and timidly began to speak.

"Hello, everybody. I'm Mollie Lewis. I'm a freshman at Vista High."

Her voice rang clearly all around the room and the loudness startled her. She pulled away from the mike instinctively as another wave of panic shook her body. What do I say now? she thought wildly.

Desperately, she looked down at her sisters for

support. Cindy was standing in the aisle behind Ken, grinning from ear to ear. Nicole was kneeling beside him, holding his hand. The two of them looked up at Mollie, their eyes glistening with pride.

In that brief moment Mollie recalled the whole succession of events that had brought her to this point. Only a few days ago she'd been totally unaware of the problems of disabled people. Her whole world had revolved around gossiping with her friends about the cutest boys at school, what to wear to the next dance or party, doing homework, having fun with her family. She'd never been involved in something this important before.

It's funny how things can change so fast, she thought to herself. An assignment from school, a book from the library, and most important, a chance collision with a guy in a wheelchair. Maybe Mollie couldn't change the world, as some of the women she'd read about had done, but she could make a difference in one person's life—and the lives of others like him.

"I'm here tonight for a very special reason," she began. In the back of the room, she could see her parents sitting side by side, beaming at their youngest daughter. She smiled and then gestured in Ken's direction.

"My friend Ken Tilson was supposed to be up here with me tonight." She giggled and waved at him.

The audience laughed, and good-naturedly Ken waved back with a grin.

"But that didn't work out," Mollie continued, her voice growing more forceful as she gained confidence. "You see, he happens to use a wheelchair to get around. And wheelchairs don't go up steps. Just because someone forgot to think ahead—or because someone thought no one would care—he wasn't allowed to share this experience with me."

The room had become completely still. Mollie paused and stared out at the audience.

"So he lost out. And I lost out, too. Because he's my friend, and I care about him."

Mollie looked down to unfold her speech. In her nervousness she'd folded it up into a tiny square. She held it in her hand for a second, then looked back out at the crowd.

"That's why I'm here tonight. I want to talk to you about caring."

With a smile she slipped her prepared text into her pocket. Mollie knew in her heart exactly what she wanted to say, and she didn't need her speech to say it.

Here's a look at what's ahead in MOLLIE IN LOVE, the twelfth book in Fawcett's "Sisters" series for GIRLS ONLY.

Unfortunately it was another day of spills and chills—Cindy, collecting more bruises than goals, became increasingly disgusted with herself. The worst part was that the Canadian boys played with disgusting fairness, so she couldn't even blame her poor performance on anyone else.

"The fact is, Lewis"—she murmured to herself, as a melee of skates and sticks sent her sprawling across the ice and into the side of the rink, where she collided with a heavy-set boy—"you're pretty lousy at this game!"

The thought did not improve her temper. Snarling at the player she had just bumped into, Cindy pulled herself back to her feet and hurried to catch up with the fast-moving play.

Mollie watched quietly with real interest from the stands. She had not accompanied Cindy and their dad to the Los Angeles Kings hockey matches and knew little about the game. It looked to her as if her headstrong sister were trying hard to get herself killed.

"Yikes, Cindy!" Mollie shrieked, watching Cindy go down yet again in a tangle of limbs and sticks.

One of the boys on the ice heard her, and skated closer to give her a reassuring smile. "She's all right; she's—how do you say—a tough acorn, your sister."

Mollie giggled. "I think you mean tough nut, but thanks for the encouragement." She narrowed her eyes a bit to study the boy more closely; beneath the bulky pads of his uniform she could tell he was tall and slender; short, dark hair framed a long, thoughtful face. A nice face, Mollie thought.

His dark brown eyes seemed to smile back at her with particular warmth. Mollie, who had plenty of practice in picking up subtle hints from the male sex, brightened at his apparent interest.

"You're very good," she told him.

The tall boy grinned shyly. *"Merci beaucoup,"* he said gravely. "I have played hockey for years."

Then a shout from the other boys drew him away, and he skated rapidly back across the rink. Mollie watched him go, almost forgetting her concern over Cindy.

It was true, she thought. He did skate with special grace, and out of all the accomplished players, this boy stood out, even to Mollie's unpracticed eyes. But it was more than his skill that kept her gaze fastened on him; it was the gentle kindness that had prompted him to reassure a worried stranger as much as the shy interest Mollie was sure she had detected during their brief conversation. She wished she had asked his name. She listened closely as the boys shouted to one another, hoping to hear someone call it out.

"Paul," Mollie murmured to herself. "I like it."

When the team called a break, several of the players drifted over to the side to get a closer look at the petite, pretty Californian who didn't seem to be as belligerent as her more athletic sister.

Mollie, delighted, smiled demurely at them all, sure that Paul would join the group, and pleased to be the center of attention. *"Bonjour,"* she said, eager to try our her scant French vocabulary. *"Je m'appelle* Mollie."

"Comment ca va, Mollie?" one of the boys, short but with wide shoulders and dancing blue eyes answered. *"Je m'appelle Raoul."*

"I'm fine, I mean, *très bien,*" Mollie answered, beginning to worry as she searched her memory for more conversation. "Do you speak English at all?"

This drew a shout of laughter. *"Mais oui,"* Raoul assured her. "We study it in school, you see."

"Good," Mollie said, sighing with relief. "My French isn't exactly perfect."

"You can say that again," Cindy observed. "You wouldn't believe what she came up with the other day at the café—"

"Cindy, don't you dare repeat that!" Mollie shrieked, forgetting to be dignified in her alarm. *That* anecdote was not one Mollie wanted floating around this good-looking group of young men!

Cindy grinned, rubbing her sore shoulder. "Relax, shrimp." She flexed her sore muscles while the rest of the boys continued to congregate around her little sister. What morons they were!

"Then you can practice your French and we will help you, yes?" Raoul suggested.

Mollie nodded. "Why were you yelling about a bird?" she asked.

"A bird?" Raoul looked blank.

"You said *'hirondelle.'* Isn't that a kind of bird?"

Another shout of laughter rose from the group.

"It's *rondelle* we were saying, *jolie* Mollie," Raoul

explained. "The hockey puck—that is what we are chasing—not a bird!"

Mollie, grinning good-naturedly at her mistake, couldn't resist a quick peek toward Paul. But he was at the outer fringe of the group, seemingly content to allow someone else to capture her attention as he examined a loose binding on one of his shin pads. Mollie felt absurdly disappointed. Had she been mistaken after all? Wasn't he interested in her?

Then he raised his head, and their eyes met. For a moment Mollie was sure that his glance was warm and eager, and she smiled. But Paul looked away again, and she felt more confused than ever.